the pilates bible

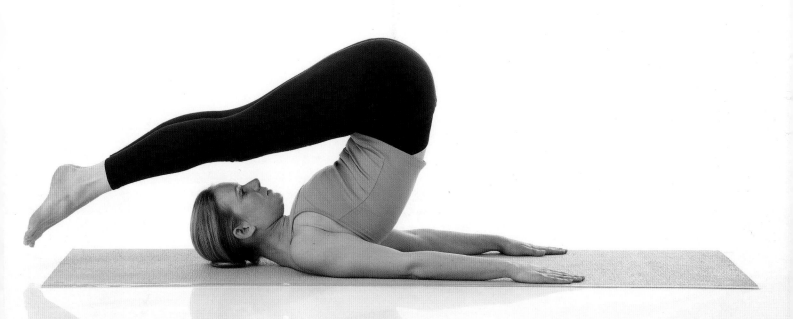

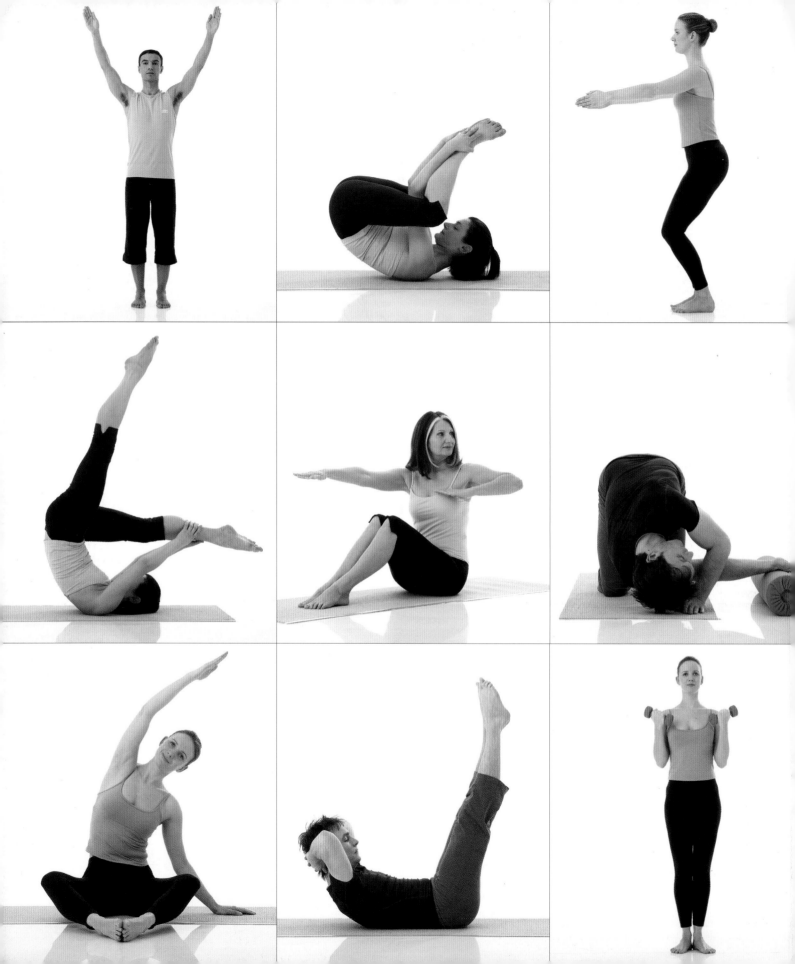

the pilates bible

bible

The most comprehensive and accessible guide to Pilates ever

Lynne Robinson, Lisa Bradshaw and Nathan Gardner

Medical Consultant: Kate Fernyhough MCSP

Kyle Books

This edition first published in Great Britain in 2011 by Kyle Books
an imprint of Kyle Cathie Ltd.
192–198 Vauxhall Bridge Road
London SW1V 1DX
general.enquiries@kylebooks.com
www.kylebooks.com

First published in Great Britain in 2009 by Kyle Cathie Ltd.

10 9

ISBN 978 1 85626 880 6

DISCLAIMER The author and publisher cannot accept any responsibility
for misadventure resulting from the practice of any of the techniques or
principles in this book. It is not intended to be and should not be used
as guidance for the treatment of serious health problems; please refer
to a medical professional if you have concerns about any aspect of your
condition or fitness level.

Project editor Katharina Hahn
Copy-editor Zoe Hughes Gough
Editorial assistant Vicki Murrell
Designer Louise Leffler
Proofreaders Maxine McCaghy and Ruth Baldwin
Indexer Alex Corrin
Photographer Eddie Macdonald
Models Marie Bartlett, Nathan Gardner, Samir Kadi, Elena Kolobkova,
Bridget Montague, Lynne Robinson
Make-up Marie Coulter (using Bobbi Brown)
Production Gemma John

Shot at Spot Studios, London, The Gym, Guildford and The Body Control
Pilates Centre, London.

Lynne Robinson, Lisa Bradshaw and Nathan Gardner are hereby
identified as the authors of this work in accordance with Section 77
of the Copyright, Designs and Patents Act 1988.

A Cataloguing in Publication record for this title is available from the
British Library.

Colour reproduction by Colourscan
Printed in China by 1010 International Printing Ltd.

Contents

Introduction

Not long before he died, in 1967, Joseph Pilates predicted that, one day, everyone in the world would have heard of his method of exercise. It took the dedication of a handful of committed clients and teachers to keep the Pilates Method alive through to the 1990s, but by the start of the new millennium, Pilates had finally exploded onto the fitness scene. Now firmly established, Pilates continues unabated in its worldwide growth.

What is it about Pilates that draws clients back to classes week after week? Perhaps it is no surprise that Pilates came to the fore around the turn of the century as people began searching for a more thoughtful way to exercise – a method that combines mental and physical conditioning and that delivers its promise of a sound mind and a strong body. From your very first session, you will feel the benefits.

'In 10 sessions you'll feel the difference, in 20 you'll see the difference, in 30 you'll have a whole new body.'

Joseph Pilates, *Return to Life through Contrology*

We are fortunate that Joseph and his wife Clara left a huge legacy of work, both on the mat and with the studio equipment. In this book, we will try to do justice to that legacy. This is no small task. There exist today many different 'schools' of Pilates. While some still adhere closely to Joseph's original work, at Body Control Pilates we have allowed his method to evolve with the times.

The legacy of Joseph Pilates

Born in Mönchengladbach, Germany, Joseph Pilates suffered from a number of serious childhood illnesses including rickets, asthma and rheumatic fever. As a result, doctors warned his parents that he would probably have a very short life expectancy. How wrong could they be! It appears that Joseph, even at a young age, had great determination. Through experimenting with many different health and fitness approaches he managed to rebuild his body strength to a fine physique.

Elements of the methods he used – yoga, martial arts, gymnastics, skiing, self-defence, dance, circus training and weight training – can be recognised in Joseph's later teaching. By selecting and absorbing the most effective aspects from each, he was able to develop a system which he believed promoted the perfect balance of strength and flexibility, and which he called 'Contrology'.

After teaching fitness and self-defence to the police and army in England, followed by an internment during World War I, Joseph returned to Germany, where he taught self-defence to the Hamburg Police and the German Army. In 1926, he decided to emigrate to the United States of America. This decision would literally change his life for, on the boat across, he met his future wife Clara and, when they realised they shared the same views on fitness, they set up a studio in New York together based on Joseph's 'Contrology' method.

For Joe, as his friends called him, and Clara the studio was a way of life rather than a business. They were more concerned with the teaching of clients than with managing the finances and they were both unbelievably generous in sharing ideas and knowledge. While the first studio clients were predominantly male – many from the boxing community – the proximity of the New York City Ballet encouraged dancers to seek Joe out when they were injured. Many of these dancers went on to become his assistants and greatly influenced the way in which his method evolved. The original exercises that Joe created were mat-based but, over time, in order to help to build the strength and flexibility of his clients and to supplement those matwork exercises, he created the various pieces of studio equipment (pages 168–193). It is a testament to his excellent design skills that the equipment used in studios today varies little from his original designs.

It was in this 8th Avenue studio that the Pilates Method as we know it today was defined. Joseph was a passionate, larger-than-life figure who ran the studio with a rod of iron. It is testament to his fitness that, despite a penchant for cigars, he lived to eighty-four years of age. He firmly believed that his method, which became known as 'Pilates' only after his death, should be part of an overall commitment to a healthy lifestyle.

Loved and respected by his clients, Joseph never doubted that one day his method of exercise would become popular worldwide – just how right he was in many of his ideas on both health and fitness makes him nothing short of a visionary. His belief in the value of self-discipline and self-help and the importance that he intuitively placed on Pilates fundamentals, such as core strength, would come to be clinically recognised in research studies carried out more than twenty years after his death.

The development of Body Control Pilates

Body Control Pilates was founded in 1995 with a vision to make the benefits of Pilates accessible to the average person, irrespective of age, income and fitness level. This represented a fundamental change from the rarefied, more studio-based approach to Pilates that predominated at that time. We saw a need for a more structured and modern approach to teaching that would meet these goals, so we created a unique programme that takes you progressively and safely towards Joseph Pilates' original work, supplemented by a comprehensive teacher training programme to enable us to build an international network of Body Control Pilates teachers. In order to do this we had to revisit Joseph's original teaching and modify many of the exercises. We see the Pilates Method not as a finite set of exercises but, rather, as an approach to mind and body training, a thoughtful movement method. In this way, we have been able to develop and grow his technique.

By drawing on the latest sports and medical research, we ensure that the Body Control Pilates approach is safe and effective. Acutely aware that our greatest teachers are both our own bodies and our own clients, we have broken down many of the original classical exercises, which are very challenging for the average person, so that they can be taught progressively. Each of our exercises will teach you a new movement skill, gradually developing your body awareness, increasing your strength and flexibility, improving your posture and coordination. Each exercise will take you one step closer to Joseph's original work. It has always been our belief that it is the quality of teaching that defines good Pilates and we are proud that Body Control Pilates is now widely seen as a benchmark for safe and effective mat and machine teaching of the highest quality. To date, we have trained more than 1200 teachers around the world.

The guiding principles

In order to practise Pilates effectively, you need to grasp the basic philosophy behind the method. Joseph Pilates taught that one of the main results of his method is gaining complete control of your body. He drew inspiration from the martial arts – slow, controlled, flowing movements performed with thoughtful awareness. Over the years, different schools of Pilates have attributed a variety of principles to the method. While these may vary in number and name, they are, in essence, the same.

At Body Control Pilates, we list eight principles that underpin our approach to the teaching and practice of Pilates:

- Concentration
- Relaxation
- Alignment
- Breathing
- Centring
- Coordination
- Flowing movements
- Stamina

Concentration

Thoughtful awareness of your whole body while you are performing the movements is key. In order to bring about change to the way you move, the body and mind need to work together. Pilates will help you to develop greater body awareness and control, through concentration and focus on the detail and precision of the exercises performed. When you are aware of the movements within each exercise, this way of moving will ultimately become automatic, bringing about unconscious improvement to the way the body moves in everyday life.

Relaxation

Relaxation of the mind and body is an essential part of any Pilates session. Focusing on releasing areas of tension within the body before, and during, each exercise is important as it allows constructive change to occur. As you focus completely on your movements, your mind feels relaxed and free from stress. It is vital to try to release unwanted tension from the body before and during the exercises. If you still hold tension, the overactive muscles that tend to dominate your movements will continue to do so. This is why you need to take time to release areas of tension at the start of your workouts. This can be done by taking a few moments going through the checklist for The Relaxation Position (page 14) or any of the Starting Positions.

Alignment (precision of movement)

Correct alignment at the start of and throughout the movement is absolutely essential. By correctly aligning the body and bringing the joints and soft tissue into their natural neutral zones, sound recruitment patterns are encouraged and the joints remain healthy. This precision of movement is the key to good Pilates practice.

Breathing

Breath is the essence of life itself. It is a movement process in its own right and therefore has great bearing on the efficiency of each movement performed. Synchronising the breath to movements is a key part of Pilates. Like any other movement in Pilates, we are looking for precision and efficiency. Breathing is no different; learning how to breathe more effectively within movement helps both the mind and body to relax, recharge and focus.

Centring

Depending on your school of Pilates, this may be referred to as 'core stability' or 'using the powerhouse'. Pilates focuses on maintaining support and control of the body as movement takes place. It does so by encouraging the recruitment of deep core muscles that help to control and stabilise movement. Staying centred involves using appropriate muscles to stabilise your core. All Pilates movements stem from a strong centre. The recruitment of the muscles involved in the centring process should be both dynamic and responsive, reflecting the demands of the movement being performed.

Coordination

Each movement involved in a Pilates exercise should be performed purposefully with control. Through focusing on the quality and detail of each movement that makes up an exercise, coordination, control, mobility, strength and the overall efficiency of the whole body are improved more effectively.

Flowing movements

Pilates movements are controlled, graceful and flowing, lengthening outwards from a strong centre. Efficiency and fluidity

are pivotal to performing the exercises correctly. You will be taught how to articulate your spine through flexion, extension, side flexion and rotation, learning how to move the spine bone by bone. Similarly, you will be mobilising your joints, taking them through their normal ranges of movement. The end result is longer, leaner muscles that are stronger through their entire range.

Stamina (muscular endurance)

Pilates exercises are usually performed only for a low number of repetitions as the focus is always on quality, not quantity. As you master each exercise, you will be learning a new movement skill. When ready, you can then add more challenging exercises to your programme. These will build muscular endurance and stamina into your body.

'Physical fitness is the attainment and maintenance of a uniformly developed body with a sound mind fully capable of naturally, easily and satisfactorily performing our many and varied tasks with spontaneous zest and pleasure.'

Joseph Pilates, *Return to Life through Contrology*

How to use this book

Regardless of your Pilates experience, you should start with The Fundamentals of Pilates (page 10). This chapter contains all the basic movement skills of our approach and is the foundation on which the whole programme is built. Even if you have years of experience, we still hope that you will find this chapter informative and extremely useful. You will find that under the headings of Alignment, Breathing, Centring and Mobility there are exercises that help to illustrate these fundamental skills. Before you attempt each exercise, read it through several times. Note the aim in the tinted box at the start of each exercise, as that will give you a clear understanding of the exercise's main objectives. Take time to find the correct starting alignment as this will impact on the precision of your movements. You will find the different Starting Positions in the Alignment section on pages 14–25. Make sure that you fully understand all the movements described in the Action. If you look at the photographs that accompany them, you will see that they provide the sequence of movements. They will also give you a visual image of what you are trying to achieve. The watch points at the end offer extra tips on how to perfect your technique and avoid common pitfalls.

The programme allows you to work at your own pace and build your skills step by step. When you feel competent at the Fundamentals, you may move on to The Beginners' Matwork Programme (page 46). At the end of this section, you will find workouts of varying lengths. These sample workouts will give you an idea of how to balance a session. You will also need to create your own workouts. When you do so, please take note of the advice given in the Workouts section. For example, you will need to include all the movements of the spine (flexion, rotation, extension and side flexion). Also take time to prepare your body before you start and to wind down afterwards. Ideally, we would like you to aim for three hours of practice per week. If this is not possible, do not despair; even a little Pilates practice, providing it is done regularly, will make a huge difference.

Once you feel capable and comfortable with all the exercises in The Beginners' Matwork Programme, you can start to learn The Intermediate Matwork Programme (page 88). Some of the exercises in this section are very difficult, so take your time and be patient. It is very important that you continue to include fundamental and beginners' exercises as these will help you build your strength and flexibility and further your understanding of the technique. Sample workouts are also provided at the end of this chapter.

The Advanced Matwork Programme (page 132) is the final and most challenging series of matwork exercises. It requires a high level of core strength, coordination and flexibility. It may well take years of practice to achieve these exercises, so approach them as a progressive journey and enjoy the process. At the end of this section, you will find the Advanced Matwork Sequence (page 166), which is our interpretation of what is often referred to as the 'Full' or 'Classical' Mat. This constitutes the full mental and physical conditioning workout that Joseph Pilates originally created.

In Chapter Five, you will discover how matwork and machine work are interrelated. This section takes you through a selection of exercises for each piece of studio equipment (The Reformer, The Cadillac, The Chair and The Barrel). If you are interested in working at home with small equipment, we have included a section where you will find exercises for all levels of ability using Stretch Bands, small and large inflatable Balls, Toning Circles, Foam Rollers and Free Weights.

Recognising that Pilates enjoys a wide variety of applications, you will also find advice on how Pilates can help with common health conditions. This is not a substitute for medical advice, but rather a guideline for how Pilates can help with maintaining general health across the different stages of life.

The principles of Pilates should not be limited to your Pilates sessions, but should be integrated into your daily life. With this in mind, the closing chapter offers advice and workouts appropriate to a wide range of activities for both work and play.

Before you begin

Here is a list of the equipment you will need:
- a padded non-slip mat
- a folded towel or small flat pillow
- a plump pillow
- a stretch band of medium strength or a long stretchy scarf

Always prepare the space in which you are going to exercise by making it warm, comfortable and free from distractions. Make sure that you have enough room to move your arms and legs without knocking any ornaments off the coffee table. If you like, you can play some background music, but it should be quiet and not distracting!

You might find it helpful to check your alignment initially in a mirror.

Wear clothing that permits freedom of movement but that will also allow you to check your alignment. Barefoot is best, but you may also wear non-slip socks.

Please do not exercise if:
- you feel unwell
- you have just eaten a heavy meal
- you have been drinking alcohol
- you are in pain from injury
- you have been taking painkillers
- you are undergoing medical treatment or taking medication

Remember, it is always wise to consult your doctor before taking up a new exercise regime. For example, many of the exercises are wonderful for back-related problems, but you should always seek expert guidance first. Similarly, not all the exercises in this programme are suitable for use during pregnancy.

Whether you are new to Pilates, a regular client, an experienced teacher or a medical practitioner, you will find this book an invaluable resource.

Chapter One:
The Fundamentals
of Pilates

This chapter is arguably the most important in the book. Whether you are new to Pilates or have many years of experience, you will find these basic skills fundamental to good practice.

We have chosen to identify four key fundamentals:

Alignment
Breathing
Centring
Mobility

Alignment

Alignment is one of our key principles, but why is it so important?

When we talk about alignment, we are referring to how you position the body both when you are 'still' and when you are moving. The reason this ranks so high on our list of priorities is that, if your body is habitually out of good alignment, it places an enormous strain on your joints, ligaments and muscles and has a detrimental impact on how you move.

One of our main goals is to improve your proprioception (awareness of where your joints are in space). If you exercise without concern for the correct position of the joints, you risk injury and additional wear and tear to the joints. Furthermore, muscles have an optimal resting length from which they function best. If you have poor postural alignment this length may be altered; muscles can end up too long or too short, and either way their ability to do their job properly is affected. By placing your joints in the right position before you start an exercise and being aware of where they are while you do the exercise, you reduce the possibility of injury and stand a good chance of getting the movement right, which means your workout is going to be really effective. This, in turn, will help to improve not only your posture but also how you move on a daily basis.

In fact, posture and movement are inseparable. It is impossible to stand completely still. We may think that we are standing still but in fact our muscles and our nerves are making hundreds of small adjustments every second in response to the pull of gravity and our surroundings. Our habitual posture and how we move are affected by a wide variety of influences ranging from genetics to personal and medical history, environmental and cultural influences. To facilitate any lasting changes to posture and movement patterns, you must understand and experience how to use your body well. This is what you will be doing when you practise the Pilates exercises in this book. You will be learning good body use as you experience good posture through movement.

With this in mind, you will notice that for every exercise in this book there are a lot of directions on how to position your body before you start the exercise and also constant reminders throughout the exercise. Correct alignment of each and every part of the body is crucial not only to safety but also to learning good body use and how to control your movements. This was part of Joseph Pilates' teaching:

'Be certain that you have your entire body under complete mental control.'

Joseph Pilates, *Return to Life through Contrology*

To help you learn this, you will also need all the other principles of Pilates.

The neutral zones of the spine and pelvis

Many of the exercises require you to start and finish with your spine and pelvis in their natural 'neutral' positions. For some of the exercises, you may also be asked to keep the spine and pelvis 'in neutral', but for others you will be moving the spine and pelvis out of neutral. Although the neutral position of the pelvis and spine are interrelated, they are not the same thing.

Let's look first at the spine. The natural curves of the spine develop during early childhood and enable the spine to absorb some of the shock that would otherwise be transmitted up to our head when we move. The deep postural muscles of the body are, when we stand, working constantly to keep us upright. One of the benefits of doing Pilates regularly is that you strengthen these deep postural muscles. As a result, standing tall with good postural alignment becomes easier. Learning how to maintain the natural curves of the spine is a proprioceptive skill that Pilates can teach you. You need also to be aware that any change in the curve of one part of the spine will have an impact on the other curves. If you habitually sit slumped in a chair, you alter the angles of the curves of the spine, which may stress the ligaments, muscles and intervertebral discs. Eventually, pain may set in.

In the Introduction, we explained how Joseph Pilates' original teachings have been adapted and modified according to current medical knowledge. Joseph actually believed that a healthy spine was a 'straight' spine, without curves. We know now that this is not the case and have adapted our teaching accordingly. He was correct, however, in his belief that elongating the spine is important. You will find, throughout the book, directions to 'lengthen up' through the spine.

In short, we are aiming for a spine that is able to retain its natural curves, an elongated S-shape. As forces conspire to compress our spine, including gravity, poor posture and old age, we can reverse these effects by creating more space between the vertebrae. This strengthens the spine, because it is those parts of the spine where one curve meets the next that the spine is at its most vulnerable. A lengthened spine that is able to articulate freely is also important (see page 242).

The angle of the pelvis will have an impact on the curvature of the spine. If you tilt your pelvis backwards, moving the pubic bone forward and tucking your tailbone under, you will lose the hollow curve (lordosis) of your lumbar spine. If you tilt your pelvis forwards, moving the pubic bone backwards, you will increase the hollow of your lumbar spine. What we are looking for is a mid-position between these two extremes. This is the most evenly balanced position of the pelvis relative to the spine and thigh-bones. It encourages the surrounding joints and muscles to be balanced and provides us with a stable base from which to move.

When the pelvis is in neutral, the pubic bone and the prominent pelvic bones (anterior superior iliac spines) are level, which means that the pelvis is tilted neither backwards nor forwards. The prominent pelvic bones should be level with each, the waist equal in length on both sides. The Relaxation Position (page 14) and The Compass (page 16) will help you find neutral.

Neutral should eventually feel natural and comfortable; it is not a fixed point to be held at all costs! However, it may take a few weeks to maintain a neutral pelvic position as often the deep stabilising muscles are weak whilst other muscles are holding tension. If you need to, initially, you may place a folded towel under your lumbar spine when you are in the Relaxation Position to help you maintain neutral. This can be useful when you are trying exercises such as Leg Slides, Knee Folds or Knee Openings. However, you should always remove this towel for other exercises that involve moving the spine. After a few weeks, as your deep postural muscles strengthen and tense muscles release, you should not need a towel.

Whilst The Compass will help you to identify a neutral position for your pelvis and lower (lumbar) spine, we also need to find a way to help you identify the best position for head and neck (cervical spine) and also the shoulders, ribcage and upper (thoracic) spine. Chin Tucks (page 18) will help you with the head and neck position while Four-point Kneeling (page 22), The Cat (page 39) and Ribcage Closure (page 37) will assist in positioning the shoulders, ribs and upper spine.

The following exercises will help to develop your awareness of good alignment in a variety of positions. They are also used as the Starting Positions for the exercises. Please note that for many of the exercises they are also the position you should return to, with control, after the movement. This is as much part of the exercises as the main action!

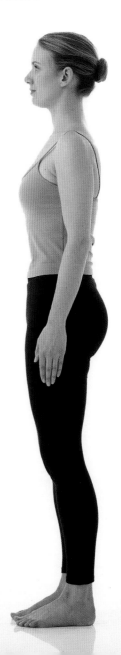

the relaxation position

A fundamental starting position offering a high level of support and providing useful feedback to alignment, making it an ideal position to start your Pilates session with.

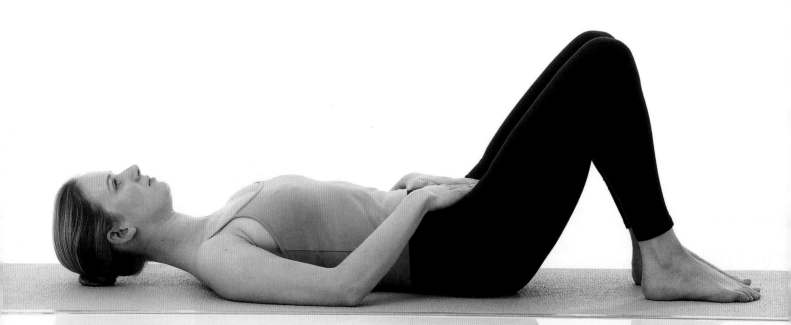

starting position

Lie on your back on a mat. Lengthen and release your neck, allowing the natural curves of your neck to be maintained; if necessary, place a small firm flat cushion or folded towel underneath your head. Bend your knees and place the soles of your feet firmly on the mat; your legs should be hip-width apart and parallel with one another.

Either:

Place the hands on your lower abdomen with your elbows bent, resting on the mat. This arm position is suitable for relaxation and awareness.

Or:

Lengthen your arms by the side of your body on the mat with your palms facing down. This arm position is in preparation for movement.

action

● Allow your entire spine to widen and lengthen as it relaxes and feels supported by the mat.

● Focus on your three areas of body weight: the back of your pelvis (sacrum); the back of your ribcage; and your head.

● Be aware of the parts of the body that are in touch with the mat and encourage them to feel heavy and supported. In your lower spine, you will feel less contact with the mat.

● Release your thighs and soften the area around the hips.

● Focus on the width across your chest and feel released in the breastbone.

● Feel lengthened in your neck and release this area, as well as your jaw and the rest of your face.

● Allow time for the body to adapt to this position and allow the spine to release.

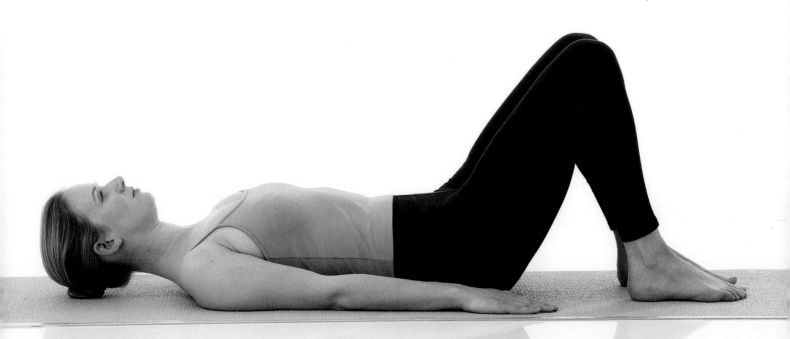

finding neutral – the compass

Helps you develop an awareness of neutral alignment around the pelvis and lower spine. Also a great way to mobilise and release the lower back.

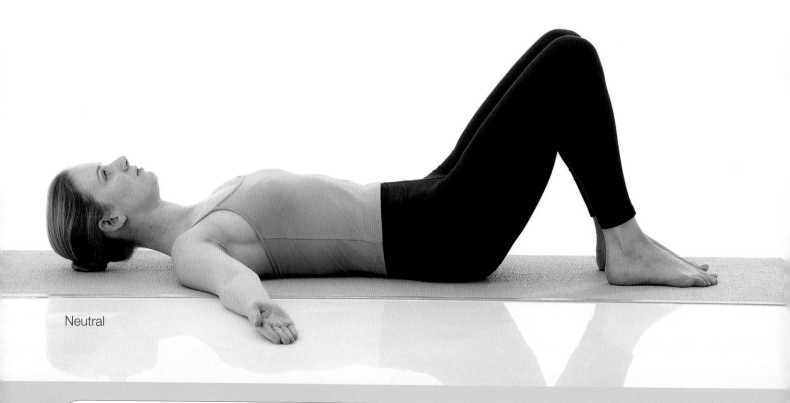

Neutral

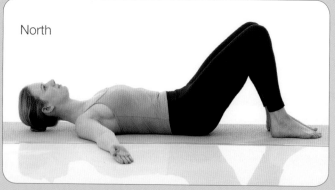

North

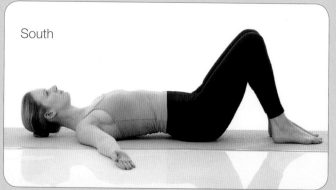

South

starting position

Align yourself correctly in the the Relaxation Position, lengthening your arms by the side of your body on the mat. Imagine that there is a compass on your lower abdomen: your navel is north, your pubic bone is south and the prominent bones of your pelvis on either side are west and east.

action

- Breathe in, preparing your body to move.
- Breathe out as you gently tilt your pelvis to the north (the pubic bone moves forwards and up). Feel your lower spine release into the mat as your pelvis tilts backwards.
- Breathe in as you tilt your pelvis back through the mid-position, without stopping, until the pelvis tilts gently forwards to the south (the pubic bone moves backwards and down). Your lower back will slightly arch.
Repeat this north-south tilt five times.
- Now, return to the Starting Position and find your neutral position, which is neither north nor south, but in between.
- Breathe out as you roll your pelvis to the west. Feel the opposite side of the pelvis lift slightly as the pelvis rotates.
- Breathe in as you roll your pelvis through the mid-position, without stopping, to the east. Feel the opposite side of your pelvis lift slightly as your pelvis rotates.
- Return to the mid-position. Your pelvis is level and this is your neutral position.

QUICK NEUTRAL CHECK
For a quick check that you are in neutral, place your hands on your lower abdomen with your fingers touching your pubic bone and the base of your thumbs resting approximately on your prominent pelvic bones to form a triangular shape. When you are in neutral, your hands are parallel to the floor and both sides of your waist are equal in length.

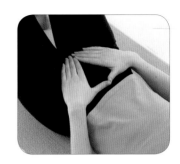

WATCH POINTS

★ The tilting of your pelvis should be small and achieved with ease. The rest of your spine will react slightly, but do not overexaggerate this.

★ The final position of neutral should feel natural and comfortable. It must not feel fixed or rigid.

★ In neutral you should feel the back of the pelvis (sacrum) heavy and grounded into the mat.

★ Allow your hip joints to be free and released.

Now we can focus more specifically on the correct alignment of the head and neck relative to the rest of our spine.

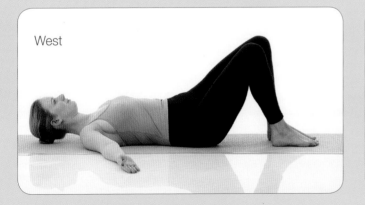
West

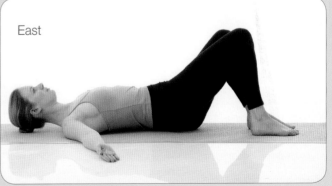
East

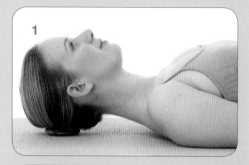

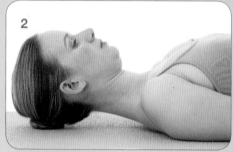

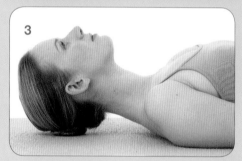

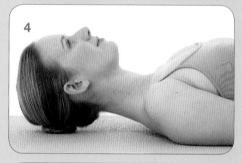

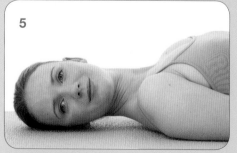

chin tucks and neck rolls

Help you develop an awareness of neutral alignment around the head and neck.

starting position

Align yourself correctly in the Relaxation Position, with your arms by your side.

action

- Breathe in, preparing your body to move.
- Breathe out as you lengthen the back of the neck, tipping your chin down. Be sure to keep your head in contact with the mat.
- Breathe in as you tip your head back gently, passing through the mid-position without stopping. Once again, keep the back of the head in contact with the mat; this is a small and subtle movement.

Repeat the Chin Tuck five times and then find the mid-position. This is neutral, with your face and your focus both directed towards the ceiling.

- Breathe out as you keep your neck released and roll your head to one side. Again, make sure that you keep your head in contact with the mat.
- Breathe in as you roll your head back to the centre.

Repeat the Neck Roll up to five times each side before returning your head to the central neutral position.

WATCH POINTS

★ The movements are very small and should feel comfortable. Be sure to perform them slowly with control.

★ Try not to disturb the natural, neutral curves of your upper and lower back.

standing alignment

starting position

Stand tall on the floor (not on your mat) and place your feet hip-width apart in a natural stance, neither turned out nor in a rigid parallel position. Allow your arms to lengthen down by the sides of your body.

action

- Lean forwards slightly from the ankle joint so that your weight shifts onto the balls of the feet; the heels stay down.
- Lean backwards slightly from the ankle joint so that your weight shifts onto the heels; the toes should be lengthened and without tension and remain in contact with the floor.
- Place your weight in the centre of the feet and notice that there is a triangle of connection with the floor: a point at the base of the big toe, the little toe and the centre of the heel.
- Lengthen your legs without bending or locking your knees.
- Tilt your pelvis forwards slightly (to the south, so that your pubic bone moves back and your lower back slightly arches).
- Then, passing through neutral, tilt your pelvis slightly backwards (to the north, so that your pubic bone moves forwards and your lower back rounds a little).
- Return your pelvis to your neutral position: a mid-position where the pubic bone is on the same plane as the prominent pelvic bones, which are also level with each other.
- Lengthen your waist equally on both sides.
- Find your centre by gently recruiting your pelvic floor and the deep abdominal muscles.
- Allow your ribcage to relax and be positioned directly above the pelvis, neither swaying backwards, nor slumping forwards.
- Feel your shoulder blades wide in the upper back, and your collarbones open in the front of the chest.
- Allow your arms to hang freely in the shoulder sockets. Feel space underneath the armpits and a sense of length and weight through the hands.
- Release your neck and allow your head to balance freely on top of the spine; sense the crown of the head lengthening up to the ceiling.
- Relax your jaw muscles and focus directly forwards.
- Whilst lengthening up, maintain a sense of what is happening in your lower body and be aware of the contact of your feet with the floor.
- Breathe naturally, this position should not feel forced or held.

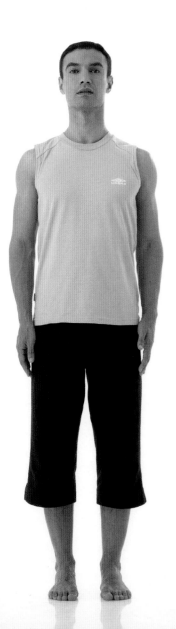
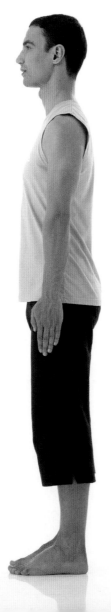

pilates stance

starting position

Stand tall on the floor (not on your mat) and slightly turn your legs out from the hips. If possible, connect your heels and place your toes slightly apart, creating a small 'V' to correspond with your legs. Connect your inner thighs. Allow your arms to lengthen down by the sides of your body.

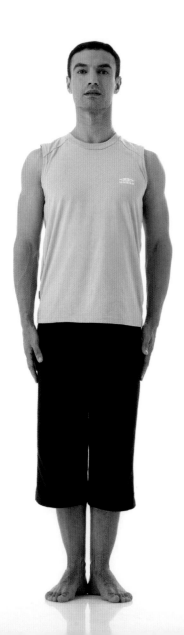

action

● Transfer your weight evenly through the soles of the feet. The toes should be lengthened and without tension.

● Do not turn your legs out too far. Focus instead on the connection of the inner thighs, the backs of the legs and an openness in the front of the pelvis.

● Slightly engage the buttock muscles, drawing them up and in, but avoid gripping, which could lead to tightness in the lower back.

● Fully lengthen your legs but avoid either bending or locking your knees.

● Balance your pelvis correctly in neutral and lengthen your spine, maintaining the natural curves of your spine.

As previously:

● Lengthen the waist, feeling equal length on both sides.

● Find your centre by gently recruiting your pelvic floor and the deep abdominal muscles for this action.

● Allow your ribcage to relax and be positioned directly above the pelvis, neither swaying backwards, nor slumping forwards.

● Feel your shoulder blades wide in the upper back, and your collarbones open in the front of the chest. Soften your breastbone.

● Allow your arms to hang freely in the shoulder sockets. Feel space underneath the armpits and a sense of length and weight through the hands.

● Release your neck and allow your head to balance freely on top of the spine; sense the crown of the head lengthening up to the ceiling.

● Relax your jaw muscles and focus directly forwards.

● Whilst lengthening up, maintain a sense of what is happening in your lower body and be aware of the contact of your feet with the floor.

● Breathe naturally into the ribcage.

● This position should not feel forced or held.

prone starting positions

A variety of prone positions is used in Pilates; the arm and leg positions vary.

starting position

Lie on your front:

Create a diamond shape with the arms: place the fingertips together, palms down on the mat, and open your elbows. Rest your forehead on the backs of your hands.

Position the legs hip-width apart and parallel.

action

● It is essential in this position, as in every other, to find the correct relationship between your pelvis, ribcage and head.

● Allow your hips to open fully and ensure that your weight is evenly distributed across the front of your pelvis. Avoid flattening or arching your lower spine.

● Your lower spine should feel lengthened. If there is any discomfort in your lower spine, you may place a very small, flat cushion or folded towel under your abdomen to help support your spine. This is a temporary solution; eventually your abdominals should be strong enough to give you the support you need. Either way, your lumbar spine should feel lengthened.

● Maintain a connection between the front of your lower ribcage and the top of your pelvis; focus on the heaviness of your ribs releasing into the mat.

● Allow your chest to be open and, although your shoulders should feel released, allow your collarbones to widen.

● Lengthen your neck whilst still maintaining the natural curve and ensure you focus directly down with your chin neither tucked in nor lifted up.

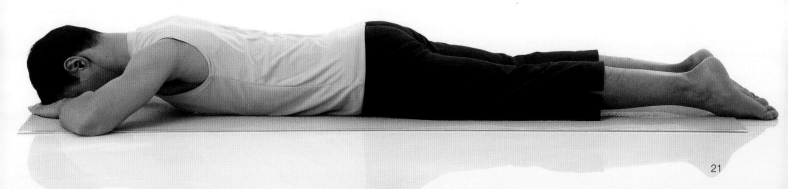

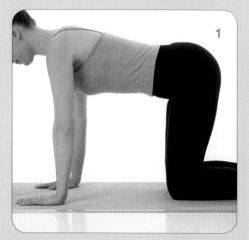

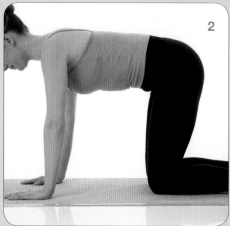

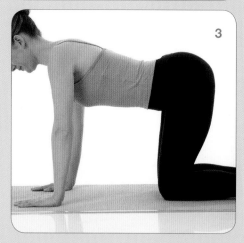

four-point kneeling

starting position

Kneel on all fours on the mat. Position your hands directly underneath your shoulders and your knees directly beneath your hips.

action

The Compass – to find the neutral position of the pelvis and lumbar spine:
● Breathe in, preparing your body to move, and lengthen your spine.
● Breathe out as you tilt your pelvis backwards (to the north – the pubic bone moves forwards), allowing your lower back to round slightly (flex).
● Breathe in, lengthening the spine, and tilt the pelvis forwards (to the south – the pubic bone moves backwards), allowing your lower back to arch slightly (extend).
Repeat three times and then find the mid-position in between these two extremes, where your pelvis is neutral. This position is lengthened and level, neither tucked nor arched.
Allow for the natural curvature of the lumbar spine.
Shoulder blade awareness – to encourage awareness of the correct position of the shoulder blades on the ribcage.
● Breathe in and, keeping your elbows straight, gently draw your shoulder blades together (retracting them). Your upper spine will slightly lower towards the mat.
● Breathe out as you allow your shoulder blades to glide wider on your ribcage. Your upper spine will round slightly.
Repeat three times and then find the mid-position of the shoulder blades in between these two extremes. Allow for the natural curvature of the upper spine and neck. Lengthen the whole spine from the crown of the head to your tailbone.

WATCH POINTS

★ In this Four-point Kneeling Position, it is essential to maintain a good abdominal connection to avoid your pelvis and spine collapsing down towards the mat.

★ The tilting of your pelvis should be small and achieved with ease. The rest of your spine will react slightly, but do not overexaggerate this.

★ Although the movements should be controlled, they should also feel free and released.

★ Fully lengthen your arms but avoid locking your elbows.

★ Keep your chest and the front of your shoulders open and avoid any tension in your neck area.

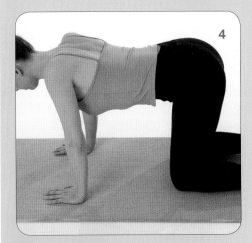

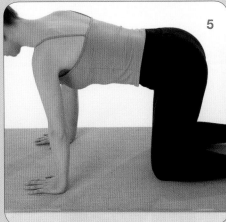

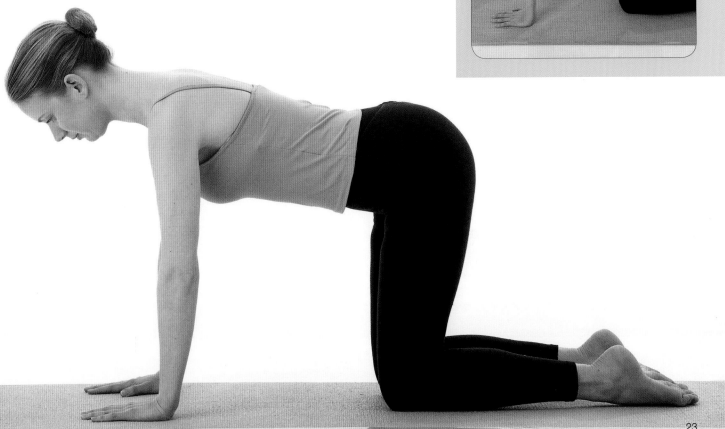

23

seated starting positions

You will find a variety of seated Starting Positions in the book. The arm and leg positions will vary.

starting position

Sit upright on the mat:

Bend your knees, turn your legs out from the hips and connect the soles of your feet.

Your feet should be quite a distance from the body to allow a feeling of space in the hip joints. Place your hands on your shins; your arms are lengthened but the elbows are slightly bent.

If you find it difficult to sit with a neutral pelvis and spine in this position, sit on a cushion or rolled-up towel to help attain the correct alignment.

action

● Ensure that your weight is balanced in the centre of your sitting bones. Neither roll too far forward arching your lower back, nor rock too far back flattening your lower back.

● Also ensure that your weight is balanced evenly between both sitting bones.

● Lengthen your spine and allow for the subtle, natural curvature of the lower spine.

● Allow your ribcage to relax and be positioned directly above the pelvis, neither swaying backwards nor slumping forwards.

● Feel your shoulder blades wide in the upper back, and your collarbones open in the front of the chest. Soften your breastbone.

● Lengthen your neck and allow your head to balance freely on top of the spine. Send your focus directly forwards.

side-lying starting positions

You will find a variety of side-lying Starting Positions in the book. The head, arm and leg positions vary.

starting position

Lie on your left side and bend both knees in front of you so that your hips and knees are bent to a right angle. To help check you are straight, line your torso up with the back edge of your mat.

action

● Some exercises require your legs to be bent, others straight. Either way, your hips should be stacked correctly one on top of the other, as should your knees, ankles and shoulders.
● Avoid your body rolling forwards or tipping back. Imagine that you are lying in between two planes of glass and stack yourself accordingly.
● Correctly align your pelvis and spine in neutral, allowing for the natural curves of the spine to be present.
● Lengthen both sides of your waist equally: this is essential in side-lying as it is very easy to allow the lower side of your spine to dip down towards the mat and for your spine to collapse.
● Ensure that your head is raised sufficiently, either supported by your outstretched arm or a cushion, to align your head and neck with your upper spine. If your head is dropped too low or raised too high, this will affect the position and movement of the rest of your body.

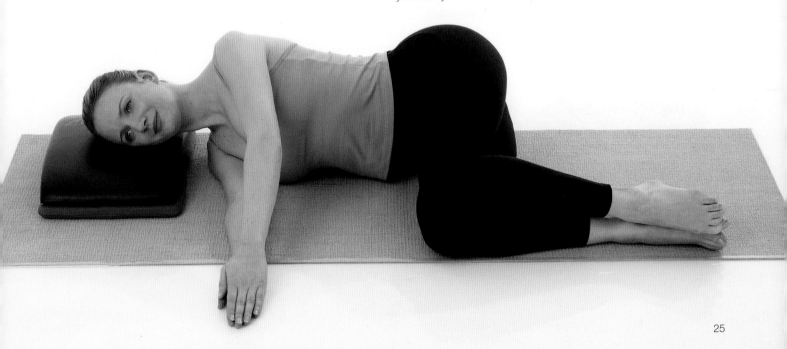

Breathing

Breathing is an automatic process that it is often ignored in our day-to-day lives. Despite the fact that breathing is vital for life, most of us are not consciously aware of it and very few of us breathe fully or effectively.

Apart from oxygenating our blood and expelling carbon dioxide from our bodies, breathing plays a very important part in movement and specifically in Pilates. It also encourages concentration, allowing us to achieve inner focus and unite the body and mind. It helps to provide a rhythm for movement and, most important, it can affect the quality of our posture and movement, which in turn helps to improve our general health and wellbeing.

According to Joseph Pilates, 'Breathing is the first act of life, and the last...above all, learn to breathe correctly.'

It may help to think of breathing as a movement process in its own right. It is not simply a static or an internal activity but one that uses many muscles, the same muscles in fact that are responsible for the maintenance of correct posture and alignment in the body. Breathing influences our actions and can help to facilitate ease of movement as well as restrict movement and create tension. Therefore careless or uncontrolled breathing can be very detrimental to our overall exercise goals.

So how should we breathe?

Lateral breathing

We need to be aware of our diaphragm, which is so essential to the act of breathing. Although you won't be able to feel it, it may help to visualise this big dome-shaped muscle separating the thoracic cavity (your ribcage) horizontally from the abdominal cavity.

First, we need to locate our lungs. They are situated towards the back of the ribcage. To help focus on this area, sit or stand tall and wrap a scarf or stretch band around the lower part of your ribs, crossing it over at the front. Hold the opposite ends of the scarf and gently pull it tight.

Inhalation

As you breathe in, focus on the back and the sides of the ribcage where your lungs are located. Like balloons swelling gradually with air, your lungs will expand and widen the walls of your ribcage. Do not be tempted to force this inhalation as you will only create tension. You should feel the scarf tightening.

It is not only the filling-up of the lungs that expands your ribcage but also the descent of the diaphragm, lowering into your abdominal area and extending outwards to a degree.

Try to breathe in through your nose and keep your shoulders relaxed.

Exhalation

To exhale means to expel the air that has been used. The deeper your exhalation, the greater your capacity to inhale new fresh air.

As you breathe out, feel the air gently being pushed out fully as if from the very bottom of your lungs and eventually exiting your body via your mouth with a deep sigh.

Your diaphragm will begin to rise and it will be easier to connect and hollow your deep abdominal muscles as you consciously empty the lungs and feel the ribcage beginning to close.

Do not puff your cheeks or purse your lips, as this will tense the neck, jaw and face and waste energy.

Remember:
- When exercising, never hold your breath.
- Breathe fully but naturally and without force.
- Breath initiates each movement and will help you to improve your flow and the enjoyable ease of your movement.
- Certain breath patterns will help particular movements, so if a movement is feeling forced or uncomfortable check first that you are breathing and second that you are breathing correctly to help facilitate the movement.

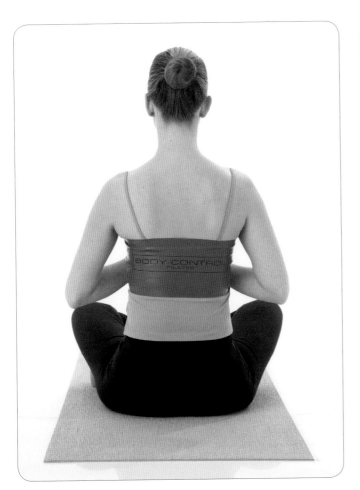

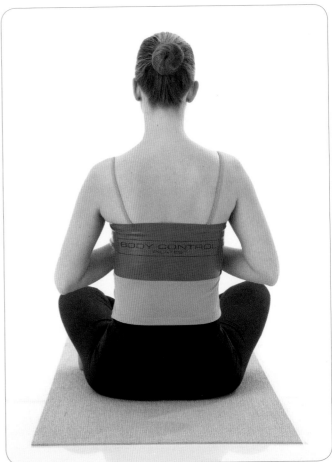

rest position

Encourages lateral breathing, providing an opportunity to refocus concentration and rebalance the spine in preparation for the next exercise.

starting position

Align yourself correctly in the Four-point Kneeling Position (page 22).

action

● Breathe in, prepare your body, lengthen your spine and bring your feet slightly closer together.

● Breathe out as you begin to fold at your hips and direct your buttocks backwards and down. Maintain the position of your hands on the mat and lengthen your arms. Ideally rest your sitting bones onto the heels, your chest onto the thighs and your forehead onto the mat.

● Breathe in and direct the breath into the back and the sides of your ribs and feel the ribcage progressively expand.

● Breathe out, fully emptying your lungs, and focus on closing the ribs down and together.

Repeat up to ten times.

To finish, breathe out and begin by rolling your pelvis underneath you and then sequentially roll and restack your spine to an upright position, sitting back onto the heels.

WATCH POINTS

★ Although this is a resting position, avoid total collapse; maintain a sense of length and activity in the position.

★ Avoid opening your knees too widely; the thighs should be slightly apart and underneath the ribcage.

★ Allow your head to be heavy and the neck lengthened and relaxed.

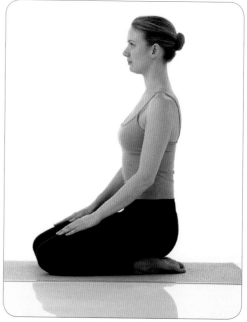

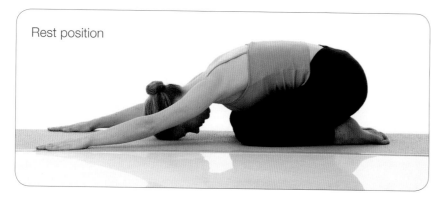

Rest position

Centring

Centring is another of our key principles and firmly underpins the Pilates method. The term 'centring' encompasses many of the popular and widely talked-about concepts associated with 'stability training'. However, the Pilates method is far more than a collection of stability training exercises.

What does 'stability' mean?

In essence, stability is about maintaining control of the movements you perform, stopping any undesired movement from occurring whilst still allowing the desired movements to be performed with maximum efficiency.

Basically, movement can occur at the various joints throughout the body. Any given movement will require some joints to move in a certain direction and sequence, while other joints are expected to stay still.

Stability is the process of stopping the joints that are not supposed to move from doing so, whilst preventing the joints that are involved in the movement from moving before they are supposed to, or from moving in the wrong direction.

The term 'centring' is just one of many used in the Pilates arena and relates more specifically to 'core stability'. Core stability is being able to stabilise and control the position of the pelvis, spine, torso, shoulders and head. Gaining stability in this core area provides a strong and stable, although not necessarily still, base of support from which all Pilates movements are initiated.

We have chosen to use the terms 'centring', 'centred' or 'centre' in this book as we feel these terms directly represent this universal key Pilates principle. It is worth noting that many other terms are also used, such as 'powerhouse', 'stabilise' and 'zip and hollow'. However, the words used are not really important, rather the feeling of the 'connection to inner control' that they convey. This connection needs to be found and maintained throughout each of the Pilates exercises being performed. In this section of the book, we focus on how to find and maintain this connection.

Connecting to your centre

Although much of the stability process is dealt with on a subconscious level, it is also possible to learn to improve stability throughout the body with conscious control. We all need stability in everyday life; this is known as functional stability. Improving your stability within a Pilates environment will help improve your functional stability on both a conscious and unconscious level.

Subconsciously, muscular recruitment for stability should be a reaction to the physical demands placed on the body. However, a certain amount of conscious recruitment can also be employed to maintain movement quality. This is especially true where the stability process is not reacting as well as it should. If you have been very inactive or injured, chances are that it isn't. In which case, it is vital that you practise all the exercises covered in this chapter before embarking on the main exercise programme. Even elite athletes need to remind themselves of these basic movement skills on a regular basis.

Do note, however, that there is a subtle balance here. Over-emphasising the stability process can lead to 'bracing' or 'fixing' which will stifle flowing efficient movement and even contribute to muscular tension. Muscular recruitment for stability should be dynamic and always relate to the challenge of the movement being performed – nothing less and nothing more than is needed to perform the exercise correctly. Think of the centring process rather like a dimmer switch that is constantly being adjusted to match the level of the demands being placed on the body.

There are many muscles involved in Centring, and most are effectively targeted by simply focusing on maintaining correct alignment while performing the exercises. In addition to this, focusing on an efficient breathing pattern and maintaining a subtle connection to the muscles around the pelvic floor and abdominal regions help to reinforce the stability process. Finding this connection to your centre can be learned relatively easily through the application of some simple cues which we will work through with the exercises in this section. Once you have mastered connecting to your centre with these exercises, you can apply what you have learned to all of the exercises in this book.

zip and abdominal hollowing

Teaches you how to feel and connect to your centre. The self-awareness that this exercise helps develop can be used in all Pilates exercises.

starting position

Sit upright on a chair. Place your feet on the floor, hip-width apart. Make sure that your weight is even on both sitting bones and that your spine is lengthened in neutral.

action

● Breathe in wide across your back and lengthen your spine.
● Breathe out as you 'zip' from the back to the front of your pelvic floor region: first, lifting from your back passage (anus) as if trying to prevent yourself from passing wind, then bringing this feeling forward towards your pubic bone as if trying to stop yourself from passing water. Continue gently to draw up these muscles inside. You should feel your abdominals begin subtly to hollow and tighten automatically.
● Continue to breathe out fully as you gently increase the hollowing of the abdominal area but do not over-engage.
● Maintain this connection and breathe normally for five breaths before releasing, ensuring that your abdominals and ribs are still able to move with your breath.

To help remind you to connect to your centre through this Zip and Abdominal Hollowing action during the exercises, you will see the following phrase repeated for each exercise: 'Maintain an appropriate level of connection to your centre throughout.'

Please remember the 'dimmer switch' (page 29) and be aware that the recruitment of these muscles should adjust according to the challenge of the exercise. The goal is to stay in control of your movements.

WATCH POINTS

★ Ensure that you do not zip, pull up, or pull in, too hard. It is very important that you do not force this action by gripping.

★ Make sure that your buttock muscles remain relaxed throughout.

★ Keep your chest and the front of your shoulders open and avoid any tension in your neck area.

★ Keep your breathing smooth and evenly paced. Ensuring that your ribcage and abdominal area are still able to expand with your in-breath is a good sign that you haven't over engaged.

★ If you lose any of the connections, relax and start again from the beginning.

★ If you find the 'zip' part too difficult, don't worry: it will come eventually. It may be easier to focus on simply scooping the abdominals, drawing them lightly back towards the spine. Above all what matters is that you are in control of your body as you move to avoid injury. This will become automatic as you practise more.

leg slides, knee openings, knee folds

Hopefully by now you are confident of how to place your body in good alignment, how to breathe laterally and how to connect to your centre. Now it is time to challenge alignment while moving by trying to control your movements from a strong centre. In the following exercises, you will be learning how to move your limbs whilst keeping the pelvis and spine still.

Below are four movements to practise, all of them requiring you to keep the pelvis completely still. You can vary which exercises you practise each session, but the Starting Position is the same for all four.

These exercises help you focus on maintaining stability between the pelvis and spine, while promoting independent movement of your leg at the hip joint.

starting position

Align yourself correctly in the Relaxation Position, lengthening your arms by the side of your body on the mat. To begin with, you may want to place your hands on your pelvis to check for unwanted movement.

preparation

- Breathe in, preparing your body to move.
- Breathe out as you gently connect to your centre by applying the Zip and Abdominal Hollowing.
- Maintain an appropriate level of connection to your centre throughout.

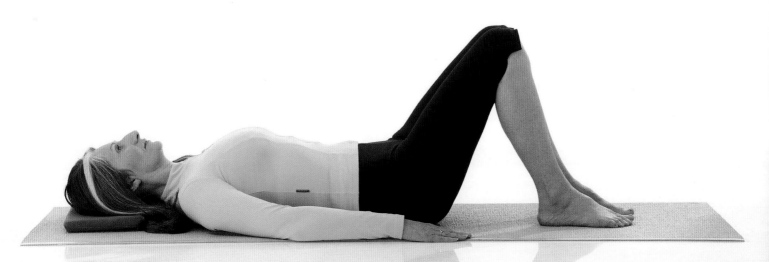

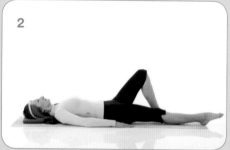

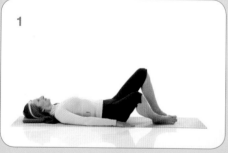

leg slides

action

- Breathe in, maintaining the connection to your centre.
- Breathe out as you slide one leg away along the floor in line with your hip, keeping your pelvis and spine stable and in neutral.
- Breathe into the back of your ribcage as you return the leg to the Starting Position; remain connected to your centre and keep your pelvis and spine stable and still.

Repeat five times with each leg.

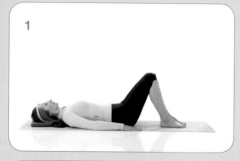

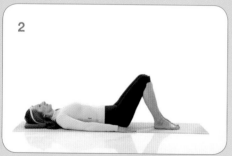

knee openings

action

- Breathe in, preparing your body to move and maintaining the connection to your centre.
- Breathe out as you allow one knee to open slowly to the side, keeping the foot down on the mat but allowing the foot to roll to its outer border. Open as far as you can without moving the pelvis.
- Breathe in as you bring the knee back to the Starting Position.

Repeat five times with each leg.

knee folds

action

● Breathe in, preparing your body to move and maintaining the connection to your centre.

● Breathe out as you lift your right foot off the mat and fold the knee up towards your body. Allow the weight of the leg to drop down into your hip socket and remain grounded in your pelvis and long in your spine.

● Breathe in, maintain the position and stay centred.

● Breathe out as you slowly return the leg back down and your foot to the mat.

Repeat five times with each leg.

WATCH POINTS

★ Keep your pelvis and spine still and centred throughout. Focus on your leg moving in isolation from the rest of your body.

★ Move your leg as far as you can without disturbing the pelvis and losing neutral.

★ Focus on your waist remaining long and even on both sides.

★ Keep your chest and the front of your shoulders open and avoid any tension in your neck area.

★ Remain still in the supporting leg, without tension.

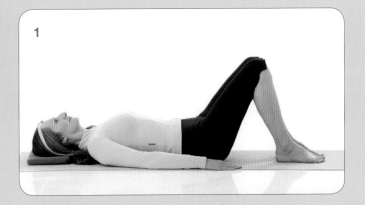

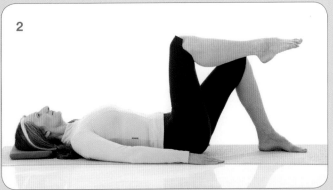

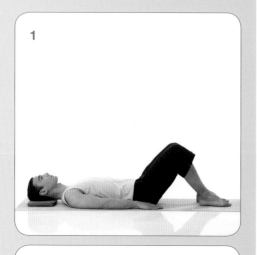

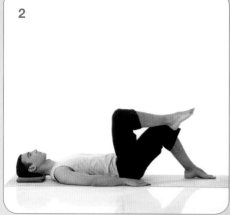

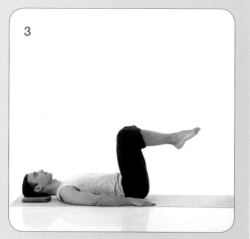

double knee folds

action

We have included Double Knee Folds here because they are a fundamental pelvic stability exercise. However, they are by no means an easy exercise to perform well and should not be attempted until you are confident with all the previous exercises in this section.

● Breathe in, preparing your body to move and maintaining the connection to your centre.

● Breathe out as you lift your right foot off the mat and fold the knee up towards your body. Remain grounded in your pelvis and long in your spine.

● Breathe in, maintain the position and stay centred.

● Breathe out as you increase your connection to your centre and fold your left knee up and towards you.

● Breathe in, maintaining your position and staying centred as your pelvis remains grounded in neutral.

● Breathe out as you slowly lower your right foot to the mat. Do not allow the abdominals to bulge or your pelvis to lose neutral.

● Breathe out as you slowly return the left leg back down and your foot to the mat. Repeat six times, alternating which leg you raise and lower first.

When you are happy that you can do this exercise easily with control, you may raise and lower each leg, still one at a time, but on a single out-breath.

WATCH POINTS

★ As for Single Knee Folds, but ensure that you use an appropriate amount of core connection, bearing in mind that lifting and lowering your second knee will require much more stability.

★ Make sure that you continue to breathe and you don't tense any unnecessary parts of your body, particularly around the neck and shoulders.

★ Fold your knees in directly in line with your hip joints.

spine curls

Promote sequential mobilisation of the spine and hips, while strengthening the back, abdominals, buttocks and the backs of the legs.

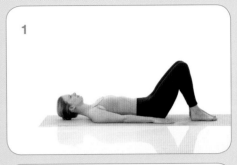

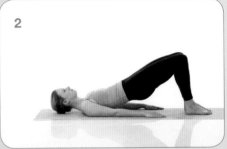

starting position

Align yourself correctly in the Relaxation Position, lengthening your arms by the side of your body on the mat.

Maintain an appropriate level of connection to your centre throughout.

action

- Breathe in, preparing your body to move.
- Breathe out as you curl your pelvis underneath you, imprinting your lower back into the mat before beginning to wheel it off the mat one vertebra at a time. Roll your spine sequentially up from the mat to the tips of the shoulder blades.
- Breathe in and hold this position, focusing on the length in your spine.
- Breathe out as you roll the spine back down, softening the breastbone and wheeling once again carefully through each section.
- Breathe in as you release the pelvis back to a neutral position.

Repeat up to ten times.

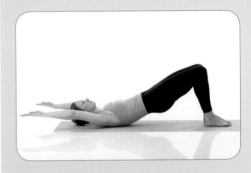

Progression: Spine Curls with Arms

Once you have mastered this exercise try floating your arms over your head at the top of the Spine Curl position and return them to your sides once your spine has returned to the Starting Position.

WATCH POINTS

★ Focus on wheeling your spine off the mat vertebra by vertebra.

★ Control the sequential return of your spine back down to the mat.

★ Avoid rolling up too far, maintain the connection of your ribs to your pelvis and avoid arching your spine.

★ Ensure there is equal weight through both feet; this will help to prevent your pelvis dipping to either side.

★ Try to avoid 'hitching' your pelvis up towards your ribcage.

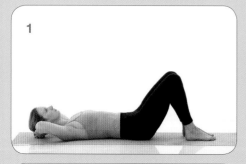

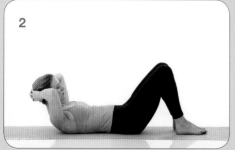

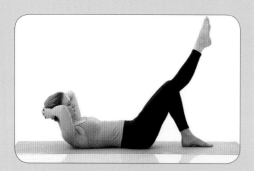

Progression: Curl Ups and Leg Reaches

Once you have mastered this exercise, try starting with your legs together and straightening one knee during each curling-up movement – then, bending it to return your foot to the floor as your torso and head return to the mat.

curl ups

Strengthen the abdominals, using them to mobilise the spine and ribcage while encouraging stability in the pelvis and legs.

starting position

Align yourself correctly in the Relaxation Position. Lightly clasp both hands behind your head, keeping the elbows open and positioned just in front of your ears, within your peripheral vision.

Maintain an appropriate level of connection to your centre throughout.

action

- Breathe in, preparing your body to move.
- Breathe out as you lengthen the back of your neck and nod your head and sequentially curl up the upper body, keeping the back of your lower ribcage in contact with the mat. Keep your pelvis still and level and do not allow your abdominals to bulge. Also, keep your head heavy in your hands.
- Breathe in to the back of your ribcage and maintain the curled-up position.
- Breathe out as you slowly and sequentially roll the spine back down to the mat with control.

Repeat up to ten times.

WATCH POINTS

★ Ensure that your pelvis remains grounded in neutral throughout; curl up only as far as this can be maintained.

★ Although your pelvis remains still, it is essential that the natural curve in your lower spine opens out and releases into the mat; you must not hold this curve.

★ Focus on wheeling your spine off the mat vertebra by vertebra.

ribcage closure

Builds awareness of spinal stability while promoting mobility of your shoulders.

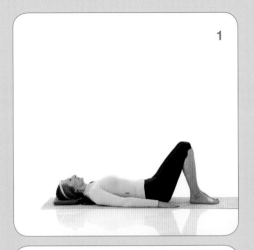

starting position

Align yourself correctly in the Relaxation Position.
Maintain an appropriate level of connection to your centre throughout.

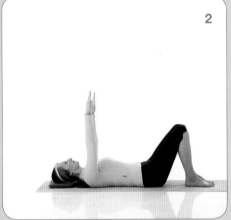

action

● Breathe in and raise both arms to a vertical position above your chest, palms facing forwards.
● Breathe out. Maintaining a stable and still spine, reach both arms overhead towards the floor. Keep your neck long and encourage the softening and the closing of the ribcage during this exhalation.
● Breathe in as you return the arms above your chest. Feel your ribcage heavy and your chest open.
● Breathe out and lower the arms, returning them to the mat and lengthening them by the sides of your body.
Repeat up to ten times.

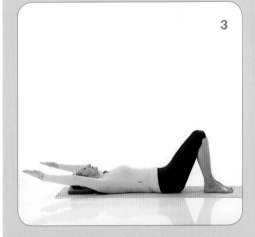

WATCH POINTS

★ Keep your pelvis and spine stable and still throughout. Be particularly careful not to allow your upper spine to arch as you reach your arms overhead.

★ Although your shoulder blades will naturally glide upwards on the back of your ribcage as your arms rise, do not over-elevate your shoulders. It is equally as important not to depress your shoulders down your back; simply allow them to move naturally and without tension.

★ Fully lengthen your arms but avoid locking your elbows.

★ Keep your neck long and free from tension.

Mobility

Mobility is directly related to stability. We cannot consider one without the other; maintaining stability of over-mobile joints is key to encouraging the less mobile joints to be more mobile.

When relaxing, we are trying to let go of unwanted tension and restriction in areas of over-activity. This forms part of the release process in Pilates. Release can also be achieved by actively lengthening the muscles by fully mobilising the joints that they cross. In Pilates, this is always an active process. Although this could be considered as 'stretching', we prefer to think of it as 'active mobilisation', as stretching is often a passive process.

Pilates improves mobility by establishing sound movement patterns rather than simply stretching tight muscles. We must always consider why a muscle is tight; it could be that there is a faulty recruitment pattern or a lack of stability around a joint. In such cases, passive stretching could actually do more harm than good. It is also important never to force the joint beyond its range of movement or to collapse or relax into the end of the joint range.

Joseph Pilates incorporated stretching into his Classical Full Mat Sequence by using one muscle group to stretch the opposing muscle group. This is a functional, safe and effective type of stretching. We should therefore consider all Pilates exercises as having a mobilisation benefit. Try to consider this with the exercises you have covered so far and in particular with the exercises in the following section on spinal articulation.

Articulation of the spine

Joseph Pilates wanted our spines to move in a 'synchronous and smooth manner' (*Return to Life through Contrology*). We have already seen how important the natural curvature is to the health of the spine and also how we want to elongate the spine to reverse any compression caused by our daily activities. We are also aiming for a spine that is both stable and mobile, a spine that can articulate freely, moving vertebra by vertebra in what is often referred to as segmental control. Although there is very little movement between adjacent vertebra, it is vital to maintain this subtle movement. The total combined movement along the length of the spine allows for an almost snakelike movement.

In order to go about our normal daily activities, we need to be able to bend forwards (spinal flexion), backwards (spinal extension), to the side (spinal lateral flexion) and to twist (spinal rotation). Pilates exercises will help you learn how to control and articulate your spine segment by segment, bone by bone, through these various movements. It is important that when you are planning your workouts, you should include all these movements.

Let's look at each in more detail.

Spinal flexion

The spine can move into flexion from either end.

In a Curl Up (page 36), you initiate the movement into flexion by nodding the head, then flexing through the neck (cervical spine) and then through the upper (thoracic) spine. With Spine Curls, you move into flexion from the opposite end of the spine by curling the tailbone (coccyx) under; the pelvis tilts posteriorly and the lower (lumbar) spine moves into flexion. With the C-Curve (page 40) the spine moves into flexion simultaneously from both ends.

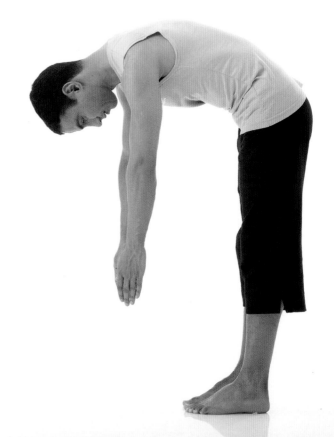

the cat

Develops mobility and release throughout the entire length of the spine while reducing pressure on the spine.

starting position

Align yourself correctly in the Four-point Kneeling Position (page 22).
Maintain an appropriate level of connection to your centre throughout.

action

● Breathe in, preparing your body to move, and lengthen your spine.
● Breathe out as you roll your pelvis underneath you, as if directing your tailbone between your legs; as you do so, your lower back will gently round and flex. Continue this flexion and allow your upper back to round gradually, followed by your neck, and finally nod your head slightly forwards. This position is a C-Curve, an even and balanced C-shape of the spine; it occurs in many of the following exercises.
● Breathe in wide to the lower ribcage to help maintain this lengthened C-Curve.

● Breathe out as you simultaneously start to unravel the spine, sending the tailbone away from you, bringing the pelvis back to neutral as you also lengthen the head and upper spine back to the starting neutral position.
Repeat up to ten times.

WATCH POINTS

★ Aim for an elongated C-Curve, which is evenly flexed throughout the spine. A common mistake is to round the upper back too much.

★ Similarly ensure that you do not over-round the shoulders. Maintain the distance between your ears and shoulders.

★ Keep the head following the same curved line of the spine; do not drop it down too far.

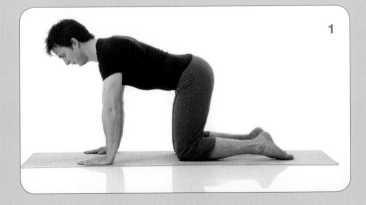
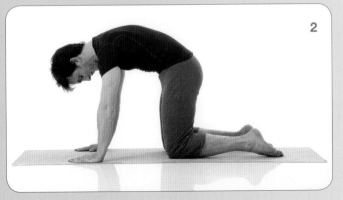

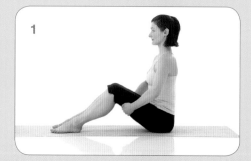

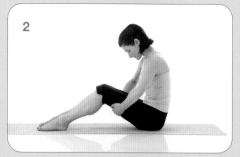

seated c-curve

Helps build an understanding of the C-Curve alignment of the spine while challenging your ability to work outwardly from a strong centre.

starting position

Sit upright with your knees bent and the soles of your feet on the mat. Your legs are hip-width apart and your pelvis and spine are in neutral. Place your hands behind your thighs with slightly bent and wide elbows.

If you find it difficult to sit with a neutral pelvis and spine in this position, sit on a cushion or rolled-up towel to help attain the correct alignment.

Maintain an appropriate level of connection to your centre throughout.

action

● Breathe in as you roll your pelvis backwards by curling your lower spine underneath you. At the same time, curl your head, neck and upper back forwards, creating a lengthened and equally curved spine. Your shoulders should remain vertically over your hips. The shape created with the spine is known as a 'C-Curve'.
● Breathe out and, moving the pelvis and head simultaneously, lengthen your spine back to neutral.

Repeat up to five times.

WATCH POINTS

★ The C-Curve is a lengthened position – avoid any compression and feel support from the abdominals.

★ Encourage an equal amount of flexion throughout the entire length of your spine. Particularly avoid any excessive bending or compression of the neck and head.

★ As your spine lengthens into the C-Curve, allow your elbows to bend slightly more, directing them out to the side.

★ Allow your shoulders to open naturally across the back while maintaining distance between the ears and the shoulders.

Spinal extension

This is the opposite movement to spinal flexion. There are many exercises in this programme that involve the spine moving into extension, but perhaps the best example is Cobra Prep.

cobra prep

Helps develop spinal mobility in and around the upper back in preparation for the full version (page 114).

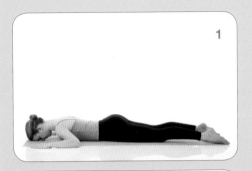

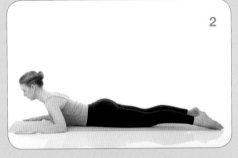

starting position

Lie on your front, correctly aligning your pelvis and spine in neutral, and rest your forehead on the mat. Your legs are straight, slightly wider apart than hip-width and turned out from the hips. Bend your elbows and position your hands slightly wider than and above your shoulders, your palms are facing down. Make sure that your shoulders are released and your collarbones are wide.
Maintain an appropriate level of connection to your centre throughout.

action

● Breathe in, preparing your body to move.
● Breathe out as you begin to lengthen the front of the neck to roll and lift your head and then your chest off the mat. Your arms will begin to straighten slightly. Feel your lower ribs remaining in contact with the mat, but open your chest and focus on directing it forwards.
● Breathe in as you hold this lengthened and lifted position.
● Breathe out as you return your chest and head sequentially back down to the mat, allowing the arms to bend back to the Starting Position.
Repeat up to ten times.

WATCH POINTS

★ Initiate the back extension by lengthening and lifting your head first, and then your neck.

★ Keep your lower ribs in contact with the mat as you lift up; this will ensure that you don't lift too far and compress your lower spine.

★ To ensure further that there is no compression or shortening of your lower spine, keep your abdominals gently connected.

★ Avoid too much pressure down into the arms; they are there to support you lightly and not to press you up.

★ Return back down to the mat with length and control.

Spinal rotation

This movement is vital to the health of the spine as it is one of the first movements to diminish with old age.

In Waist Twists, focus on sequential rotation; initiate the movement by first turning your head and then your neck and your upper spine follow. There is a minimal amount of rotation in the lower spine because the pelvis stays still. Maintain length in your spine and focus on connecting to your centre throughout.

waist twist

Works the muscles around your waist while promoting spinal mobility with a balanced rotation of the head, neck and torso.

starting position

This exercise can be performed sitting or standing.
Either:
Sit upright with your legs bent and turned out, and the soles of your feet connected. Your feet should be quite a distance from the body to allow a feeling of space in the hip joints. Your pelvis and spine are in neutral. Fold your arms in front of your chest, just below shoulder height. One palm is on top of the opposite elbow and the other hand is positioned underneath the opposite elbow. If you find it difficult to sit with a neutral pelvis and spine in this position, sit on a cushion or rolled-up towel to help attain the correct alignment. (This exercise may also be performed seated on a chair, feet placed hip-width apart on the floor.)
Or:
Stand tall on the floor (not on your mat) and lengthen your spine into neutral. Your legs are in parallel and hip-width apart. Position your arms as for sitting.
Maintain an appropriate level of connection to your centre throughout.

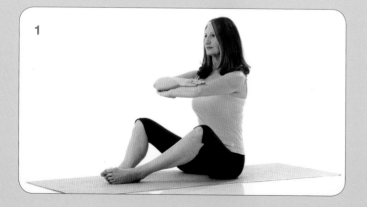

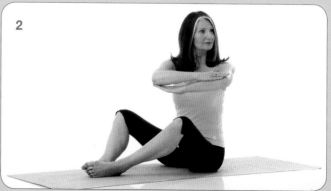

action

- Breathe in, preparing your body to move, and lengthen your spine.
- Breathe out as you initiate with a turn of the head and rotate your torso fully to the left. Keep your pelvis stable and keep lengthening up through the crown of the head.
- Breathe in as you continue to lengthen your spine and rotate back to the Starting Position.

Repeat five times to each side.

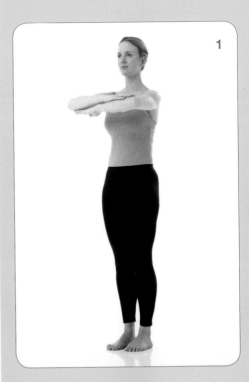

WATCH POINTS

★ Your pelvis should remain still. Keep the weight even on either your sitting bones or your feet (depending on your Starting Position) and maintain their contact to the mat/floor throughout.

★ Focus on engaging your deep abdominals to help support your spine as you rotate and return.

★ The movement is pure rotation. Continue to keep the spine lengthening vertically and avoid arching in your back or shortening in your waist.

★ Carry your arms with the spine; do not allow them to lead the movement.

★ Allow maximum rotation of the head and neck, but ensure length throughout.

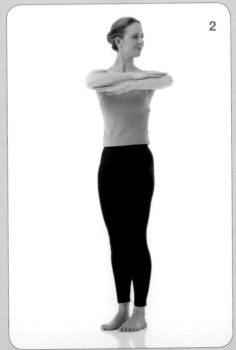

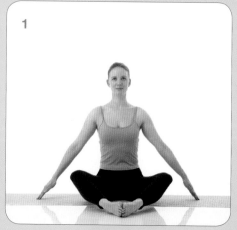

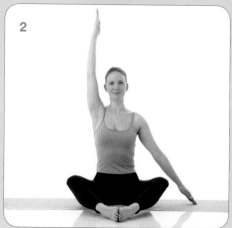

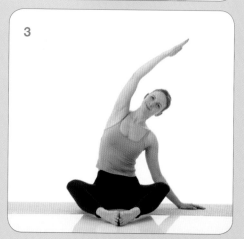

Spinal lateral flexion

As you bend to the side, your spine moves into lateral flexion. Ideally we want to encourage sequential lateral flexion. As you reach over, initiate the movement with an incline of your head and continue moving through your neck and then your ribcage. Reverse the sequence as you return to the upright position, always maintaining length in your spine and focusing on the connection to your centre.

side reach

Promotes release along the sides of the body by mobilising the spine in a sideways-bending motion. This is often an area of hidden tension in the body which really benefits from being moved in this way.

starting position

Again, this exercise can be performed either sitting or standing.
Either:
Sit upright with your legs bent and turned out, and the soles of your feet connected.
Your feet should be quite a distance from the body to allow a feeling of space in the hip joints. Your pelvis and spine are in neutral. Allow your arms to lengthen down by the sides of your body.
If you find it difficult to sit with a neutral pelvis and spine in this position, sit on a cushion or rolled-up towel to help attain the correct alignment. (This exercise may also be performed seated on a chair, feet placed hip-width apart on the floor.)
Stand tall on the floor (not on your mat) and lengthen your spine into neutral. Your legs are in parallel and hip-width apart. Allow your arms to lengthen down by the sides of your body.
Maintain an appropriate level of connection to your centre throughout.

action

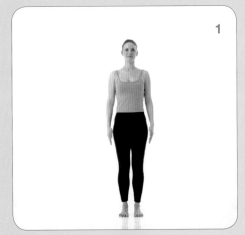

- Breathe in as you raise your right arm out to the side and overhead.
- Breathe out as you reach up and over, leading with your head, sequentially bending your spine to the left. Maintain the relationship between the right arm and your head. If sitting, your left arm will reactively slide further along the mat and then bend, so that your forearm can support your position. If standing, your left arm will remain lengthened and slide down the outside of your left leg.
- Breathe in. Maintain the length and position of your spine and focus on breathing laterally.
- Breathe out as you return the spine back to the vertical position. Lower your right arm down by your side.

Repeat five times to each side.

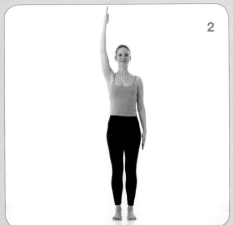

WATCH POINTS

★ As you side-bend, initiate the movement with your head, followed sequentially by your ribcage. As you return, initiate the movement from your centre.

★ The side bend should be a lengthened position; avoid any compression and feel support from the abdominals.

★ Ensure that you have moved in one plane only and not curved forward or arched back.

★ Maintain openness across your chest and the back of your shoulders, avoiding over reaching with your arms. Keep a relationship between the shoulders and the back of your ribcage; neither force them to depress, nor allow them to over-elevate.

★ Keep your shoulders and neck free from tension throughout.

★ Keep your head and neck in line with the rest of your spine.

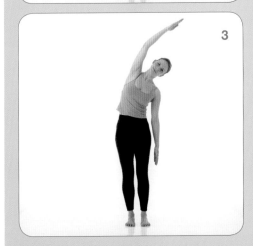

Combined movements

The exercises above have demonstrated the spine moving into pure flexion, extension, rotation and lateral flexion. You will need to learn how to do these slowly with control. Once this is mastered, you can start to include exercises that have combined movements, for example Oblique Curls and Saw, which involve flexion and rotation of the spine. Many of the exercises in the Advanced Programme (page 132) involve complex combinations.

Chapter Two:
The Beginners' Matwork Programme

What follows is a selection of Pilates matwork exercises that are suitable for anyone new to Pilates, or for those wishing to review good movement skills before continuing with more advanced work. Once you have understood the fundamentals in the previous chapter, and established a sense of correct alignment, centring and breathing, feel free to move on to our beginners' exercises.

All of the exercises clearly explain their individual aim, but do bear in mind that all Pilates exercises work to utilise the entire body. Each exercise, no matter how specific it may seem, will in some way be suitable for you and your body.

To help you to group together a balanced selection of exercises that fits into your day, we have created Beginners' Workouts of different lengths (page 86).

the exercises

1. Shoulder Drops
2. Arm Circles
3. Pelvic Clocks
4. Windows
5. Knee Circles
6. Oblique Curl Ups
7. Hip Rolls
8. Floating Arms
9. Table Top
10. Diamond Press

11. Dart
12. Bow and Arrow – Sitting
13. Bow and Arrow – Lying
14. Arm Openings
15. Tennis Ball Rising
16. Single Leg Stretch – Preparation
17. Double Leg Stretch – Preparation
18. Knee Rolls
19. Oyster
20. Zigzags – Lying

21. Zigzags – Sitting
22. Creeping Feet
23. Mexican Wave
24. Ankle Circles
25. Standing on One Leg
26. Pilates Squats
27. Wrist Circles
28. Dumb Waiter
29. Roll Downs – Against a Wall
30. Roll Downs – Freestanding

shoulder drops

Help release tension from around the shoulders and neck by mobilising the shoulder blades. Also helps develop awareness of the arms' connection to the back of the ribcage.

starting position

Align yourself correctly in the Relaxation Position. Raise both arms vertically above your chest, shoulder-width apart, palms facing one another.

Maintain an appropriate level of connection to your centre throughout.

action

● Breathe in as you reach one arm up towards the ceiling, peeling the shoulder blade away from the mat.
● Breathe out as you gently release the arm back down, returning the shoulder blade back onto the mat.
Repeat up to ten times, alternating arms.

Variation

Reach and release both arms at the same time.

WATCH POINTS

★ Keep your pelvis and spine stable and still throughout.

★ Keep your neck long and free from tension; your head remains still and heavy throughout.

★ Use the breathing pattern to guide your movements: the inhalation encourages the ribcage to widen and the shoulder blades to glide; the exhalation encourages a release of tension.

★ Fully lengthen your arms but avoid locking your elbows.

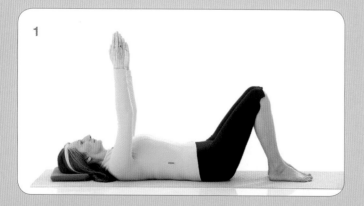

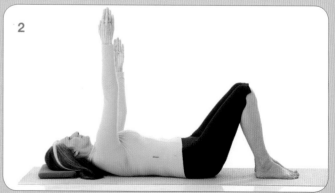

arm circles

Helps to mobilise the chest and shoulder area while challenging the stability of the spine.

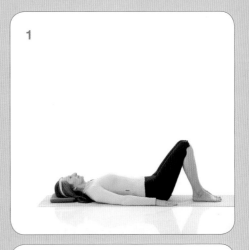

starting position

Align yourself correctly in the Relaxation Position, lengthening your arms by the side of your body on the mat.

Maintain an appropriate level of connection to your centre throughout.

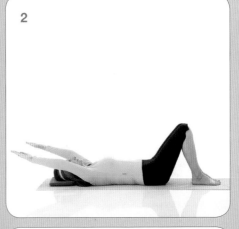

action

- Breathe in, preparing your body to move.
- Breathe out as you raise both arms above the chest, and then reach them overhead towards the mat. Focus on softly closing down the ribcage as you exhale.
- Breathe in as you circle your arms out to the side and down towards the body. As the arms return to the starting position, turn your palms to the mat. Repeat up to five times and then reverse the direction.

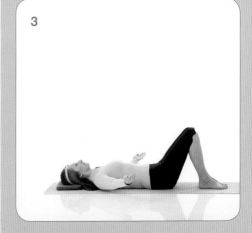

WATCH POINTS

★ Keep your pelvis and spine stable and still throughout. Be particularly careful not to allow your upper spine to arch as you reach your arms overhead.

★ Although your shoulder blades will naturally glide upwards on the back of your ribcage as your arms rise, do not over-elevate your shoulders. It is equally as important not to depress your shoulders down your back; simply allow them to move naturally and without tension.

★ Fully lengthen your arms but avoid locking your elbows.

★ As the arms circle, keep them on the same plane to help maintain openness in the front of the shoulder joints.

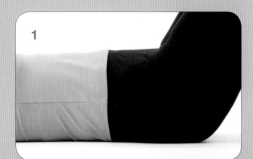

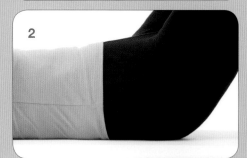

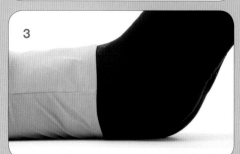

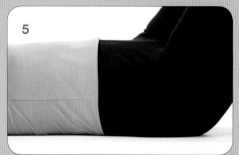

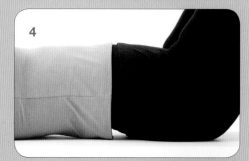

pelvic clocks

Develop an awareness of neutral alignment around the pelvis and lower spine while mobilising the lower back and hips.

starting position

Align yourself correctly in the Relaxation Position. Imagine that there is a clock face on your lower abdomen – your navel is twelve o'clock, your pubic bone six o'clock, and your prominent pelvic bones are three o'clock and nine o'clock on either side. Visualise a marble in the middle of the clock face.

Maintain an appropriate level of connection to your centre throughout.

action

- Breathe in, preparing your body to move.
- Breathe out as you gently tilt your pelvis and visualise rolling the marble to twelve o'clock. Feel your lower spine release into the mat. Continue to roll the marble around to one o'clock and so on, rotating your pelvis until arriving at six o'clock where the pelvis will be centred and tilted forwards slightly. Feel your lower back gently arch.
- Breathe in and continue to roll the marble around and up to seven o'clock and so on, rotating the pelvis until arriving in the centre once again at twelve o'clock. Your pelvis is tilted back slightly and your lower spine is once again imprinting gently into the mat. Repeat up to five times and reverse direction.

WATCH POINTS

★ The tilting and rolling of your pelvis should be small and achieved with ease. The rest of your spine will react slightly, but do not over-exaggerate this.

★ Ensure that your waist remains equally lengthened on both sides. Try to avoid 'hitching' your pelvis up towards your ribcage as you roll.

windows

Open the front of the shoulders and chest by moving the arms with well-ordered movement in the shoulders; challenges spinal stability.

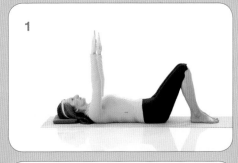

starting position

Align yourself correctly in the Relaxation Position. Raise both arms vertically above your chest, shoulder-width apart, with your palms facing forwards.
Maintain an appropriate level of connection to your centre throughout.

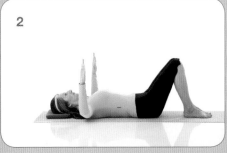

action

- Breathe in, preparing your body to move.
- Breathe out as you bend both elbows, directing them down towards the mat. Keep the elbows in line with your shoulders. Depending on your flexibility and range of movement, your arms may or may not touch the mat.
- Breathe in as you rotate the arms, lowering the forearms and the backs of your hands towards the mat.
- Breathe out as you straighten the arms, reaching them overhead.
- Breathe in as you return both arms above your chest and back to the Starting Position. Repeat up to ten times.

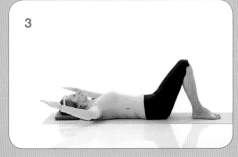

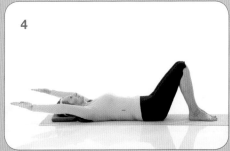

WATCH POINTS

★   Keep your pelvis and spine stable and still throughout.

★   Although your shoulder blades will glide naturally upwards on the back of your ribcage as your arms rise, do not over-elevate your shoulders. It is equally as important not to depress your shoulders down your back; simply allow them to move naturally and without tension.

★   Try to keep your forearm and upper arm on the same plane when straightening the arms overhead.

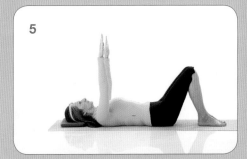

knee circles

Teach you to move your thigh bone independently from your pelvis and spine, releasing tension around the hip joint while improving spinal stability.

starting position

Align yourself correctly in the Relaxation Position. Fold one leg in towards your body with control and bend the knee further, fully relaxing the lower leg.

Maintain an appropriate level of connection to your centre throughout.

action

● Breathing naturally and, at your own pace, begin to circle your leg towards the mid-line of the body and then continue to circle the leg down, around and back up to the Starting Position. Draw your leg in as close to the body as is possible without disturbing the pelvis.

Repeat up to five times and then reverse the direction.

● To finish, return your knee so that it is in line with the hip joint and then, maintaining a stable pelvis, return your leg to the mat to finish in the Relaxation Position.

Repeat with the other leg, five times in each direction.

WATCH POINTS

★ Keep your pelvis and spine stable and still throughout; focus on the independent movement of the thigh bone in the hip socket.

★ Keep the supporting leg still, without tension.

★ Keep your chest and the front of your shoulders open and avoid any tension in your neck area.

★ Begin with small circles, about the size of a grapefruit, and work up to larger circles as you learn to gain more control.

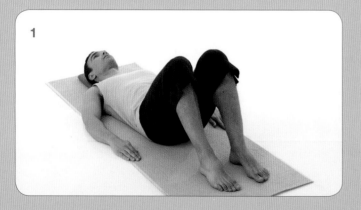

1

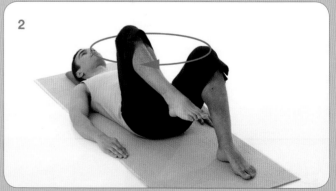

2

oblique curl ups

This exercise strengthens the abdominals, using them to mobilise the spine and ribcage, while challenging pelvic stability.

starting position

Align yourself correctly in the Relaxation Position. Lightly clasp both hands behind your head, keeping the elbows open and positioned just in front of your ears, within your peripheral vision.

Maintain an appropriate level of connection to your centre throughout.

action

- Breathe in, preparing your body to move.
- Breathe out as you nod your head and sequentially curl up the upper body, rotating your head and torso to the right and directing the left side of your ribcage towards your right hip. Keep your pelvis still and level and do not allow your abdominals to bulge.
- Breathe in to the back of your ribcage and maintain the curled and rotated position.
- Breathe out as you slowly and sequentially roll back down to the centre with control.

Repeat, this time rotating to the left. Repeat up to ten times.

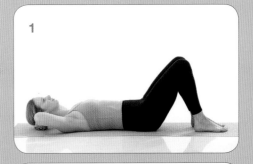

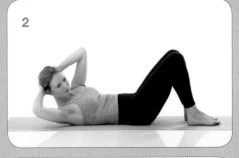

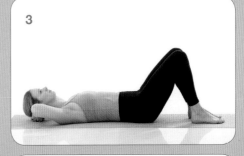

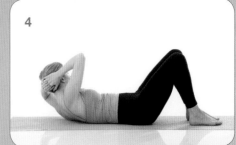

WATCH POINTS

★ Ensure that your pelvis remains grounded in neutral and square throughout; curl up only as far as this can be maintained.

★ Keep both sides of the waist equally long.

★ The rotation should come from the movement of the ribs on the spine and the spine itself. Try not to pull on your head and neck.

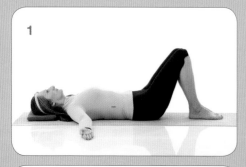

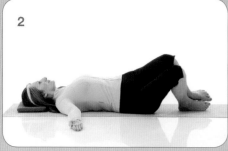

hip rolls

Challenge your ability to mobilise your waist and torso with control while maintaining stability and release across your upper body.

starting position

Align yourself correctly in the Relaxation Position. Bring your legs together and connect your inner thighs. Reach your arms out on the mat slightly lower than shoulder height with your palms facing upwards.

Maintain an appropriate level of connection to your centre throughout.

action

● Breathe in and, maintaining the connection of the inner thighs, begin to rotate your pelvis and legs to the right from a strong centre. The left side of the pelvis and the lower left ribs will peel slightly off the mat.

● Breathe out as you return the pelvis and legs back to the Starting Position, initiating from your centre.

Repeat to the other side and then repeat the whole sequence up to five times.

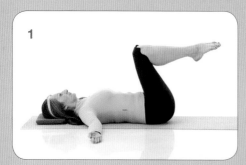

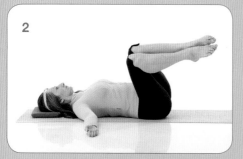

Progression: Hip Rolls – Feet Up

Once you have mastered this exercise, try bringing your legs into a Double Knee Fold position (page 34) and performing the Hip Roll action from this position.

WATCH POINTS

★ Roll your pelvis and your legs directly to the side and avoid any deviation; there should be no shortening on either side of the waist.

★ Maintain a connection between your ribcage and your pelvis and ensure that you don't arch your back as you roll.

★ Control the movement of your legs and don't just allow them to 'drop'.

★ Ensure the foot that is on top peels away from the mat during the roll.

★ Keep your chest and the front of your shoulders open and avoid any tension in your neck area.

floating arms

Mobilise the shoulder joints, promoting openness across the front of the torso.

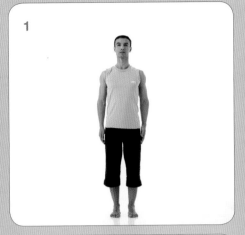

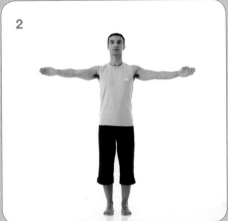

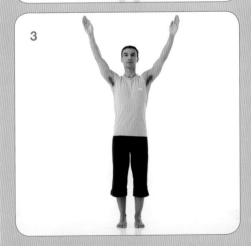

starting position

Stand tall on the floor (not on your mat) and lengthen your spine into neutral. Your legs are either parallel and hip-width apart or connected in Pilates Stance. Allow your arms to lengthen down by the sides of your body.

Maintain an appropriate level of connection to your centre throughout.

action

● Breathe in, preparing your body to move, and lengthen your spine.

● Breathe out and, keeping your arms lengthened and the spine stable, raise both arms out to the side, slightly forwards and up above your body.

● Breathe in and lower the arms slightly forwards and down on the same pathway to the side of the body.

Repeat up to ten times.

WATCH POINTS

★ Continue to maintain a stable and lengthened vertical position of your pelvis and spine throughout.

★ Although your shoulder blades will naturally glide upwards on the back of your ribcage as your arms rise, do not over-elevate your shoulders. It is equally as important not to depress your shoulders down your back; simply allow them to move naturally and without tension.

★ Use the exhalation to encourage your breastbone to soften and close the ribcage as you raise your arms upwards. Keep your chest open.

★ Without locking your elbows keep your arms lengthened and not bent. Ensure that the movement comes only from the shoulders.

table top

Challenges the stability of the entire spine and shoulder girdle while moving opposing arms and legs freely.

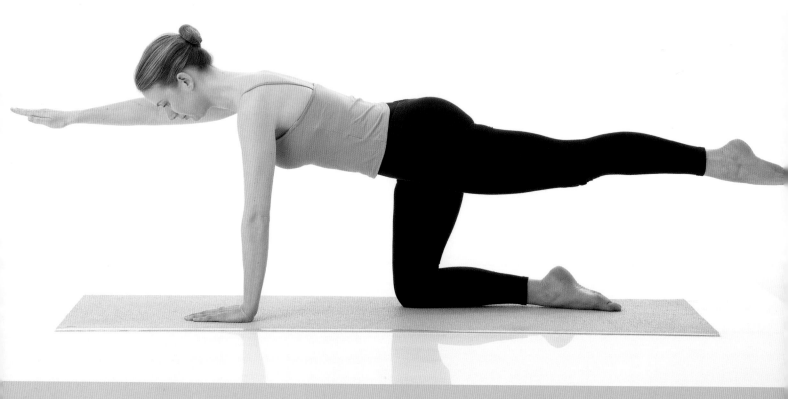

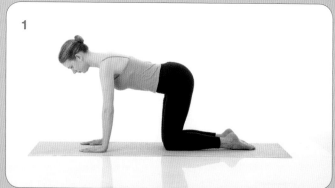

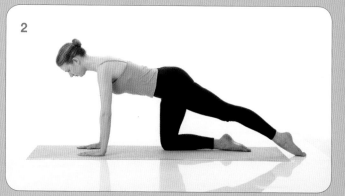

starting position

Align yourself correctly in the Four-point Kneeling Position. Maintain an appropriate level of connection to your centre throughout.

action

● Breathe in, preparing your body to move, and lengthen your spine.
● Breathe out and, maintaining a still and stable pelvis and spine, slide one leg behind you, directly in line with your hip. Your softly pointed foot will remain in contact with the mat.
● Breathe in as you lengthen and lift your leg to hip height. Simultaneously raise the opposite arm forwards, ideally to shoulder height. Again maintain a lengthened and stable torso.
● Breathe out and lower your lengthened leg to the mat, and simultaneously return your arm underneath your shoulder.
● Breathe in and, once again maintaining neutral pelvis and spine, slide your leg back to the Starting Position.
Repeat up to five times on each side, alternating the opposite arm and leg.

Variation

If you find this exercise too challenging, leave your foot in contact with the floor once your leg has straightened. This will help you maintain your balance and reduce the work in your lower back. If it is still too difficult, miss out the arm movement too and concentrate on the action of the sliding leg.

WATCH POINTS

★ In this Four-point Kneeling Position, it is essential to maintain good abdominal connection to avoid your spine dipping down towards the mat.

★ Keep lengthening both sides of the waist throughout. Try to avoid 'hitching' your pelvis up towards your ribcage.

★ Your arm should ideally rise to the height of your shoulder, your leg to the height of your hip, but lift this high only if you can maintain stillness in your pelvis and spine.

★ Although your shoulder blade will naturally glide upwards on the back of your ribcage as your arm rises, do not over-elevate your shoulder. It is equally as important not to depress your shoulder down your back; simply allow it to move naturally and without tension.

★ Correctly coordinate the timing of your arm with your leg movement.

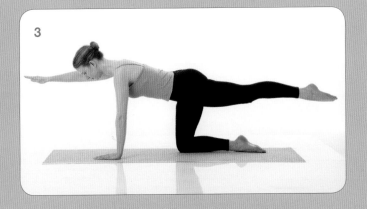

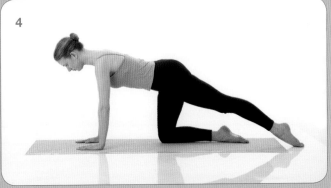

diamond press

Helps develop spinal mobility in and around the upper back, while opening across the front of the shoulders.

starting position

Lie on your front, correctly aligning your pelvis and spine in neutral. Create a diamond shape with the arms: place the fingertips together and palms down onto the mat and open your elbows. Rest your forehead on the backs of the hands. Your legs are hip-width apart and parallel.

Maintain an appropriate level of connection to your centre throughout.

action

- Breathe in, preparing your body to move.
- Breathe out as you lift first your head, then your neck and then your chest off the mat. Feel your lower ribs remaining in contact with the mat, but open your chest and direct it forwards.
- Breathe in as you hold this lengthened and stable position.
- Breathe out as you return your chest and head sequentially back down to the mat.

Repeat up to ten times.

WATCH POINTS

★ Initiate the back extension by lengthening and lifting your head first, and then your neck. When your head and neck are in line with your spine you can begin to open and lift your chest.

★ Keep your lower ribs in contact with the mat as you lift up; this will ensure that you don't lift too far and compress your lower spine. The length throughout the spine is far more important than the height of extension that you achieve.

★ Avoid too much pressure down into the arms; they are there to support you lightly and not to press you up.

★ Keep your feet in contact with the mat throughout.

★ As you return back down to the mat, do not collapse; return with length and control.

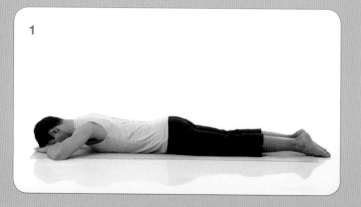

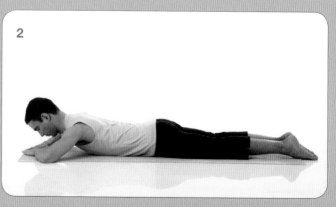

dart

Strengthens the back muscles while mobilising the upper spine and promoting the use of the inner thighs to help connect and maintain a strong centre.

starting position

Lie on your front, correctly aligning your pelvis and spine in neutral. Rest your forehead on a small cushion and lengthen your arms by the side of your body on the mat; your palms are facing the ceiling. Your legs are straight but relaxed with the base of your big toes touching.

Maintain an appropriate level of connection to your centre throughout.

WATCH POINTS

★ Initiate the back extension by lengthening and lifting your head first, and then your neck.

★ Keep the lift small to avoid compressing the spine; return down with length and control.

★ Keep your feet in contact with the mat throughout.

action

● Breathe in, preparing your body to move.

● Breathe out as you lift first your head, then your neck and then your chest and upper spine off the mat. Feel your lower ribs remaining in contact with the mat. Lengthen your arms away and lift them slightly as they turn in, palms facing your body. Simultaneously draw your legs together, connecting the inner thighs in a parallel position.

● Breathe in as you hold this lengthened and stable position, feeling the opposition of the crown of your head reaching away from your toes.

● Breathe out as you return the spine and head sequentially back down to the mat, simultaneously releasing your legs and arms back into the Starting Position.

Repeat up to ten times.

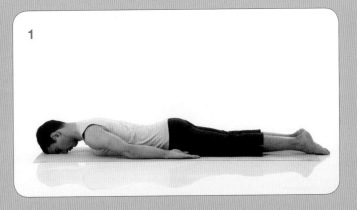

1

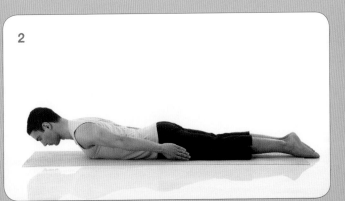

2

bow and arrow – sitting

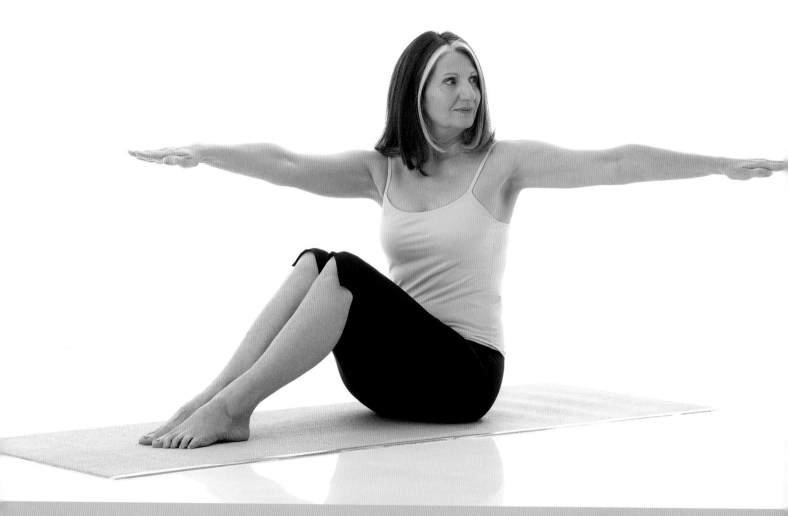

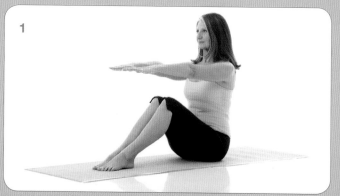

1

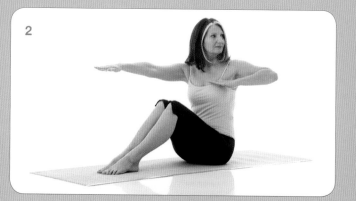

2

Promotes spinal mobility with a balanced rotation of the head, neck and torso coupled with a smooth dynamic arm movement.

starting position

Sit upright with your knees bent and the soles of your feet grounded on the mat. Your legs are together with the inner thighs connected. Your pelvis and spine are in neutral. Reach your arms out in front of you, slightly lower than shoulder height and shoulder-width apart. Your arms are lengthened, and your palms are facing down.

If you find it difficult to sit with a neutral pelvis and spine in this position, sit on a cushion or rolled-up towel to help attain the correct alignment. (This exercise may also be performed seated on a chair, with your feet placed hip-width apart on the floor.) Maintain an appropriate level of connection to your centre.

action

● Breathe in; lengthen and prepare your body to move.
● Breathe out as you bend your left elbow, drawing the arm towards your body and the left hand towards your left shoulder. Simultaneously rotate your head, neck and upper spine to the left.
● Breathe in as you straighten the left elbow. Lengthen your spine and encourage a little more rotation.
● Breathe out as you rotate the spine back, keeping the right arm straight, and return to the Starting Position.
Repeat to the other side and then repeat the whole sequence up to five times.

WATCH POINTS

★ Your pelvis should remain still. Keep the weight even on both sitting bones and maintain their contact to the mat throughout.

★ Focus on connecting your deep abdominals to help support your spine as you rotate and return.

★ The movement is pure rotation; continue to lengthen the spine vertically. Avoid arching in your back or shortening in your waist.

★ Your arms should move only as your spine moves; do not allow them to initiate the movement or move beyond the rotation of the spine.

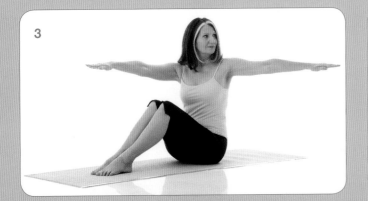

3

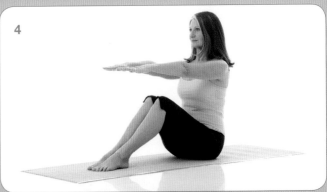

4

bow and arrow – lying

Mobilises the head, neck and torso through a balanced rotational movement coupled with a flowing arm movement that promotes control in the shoulders and openness across the chest.

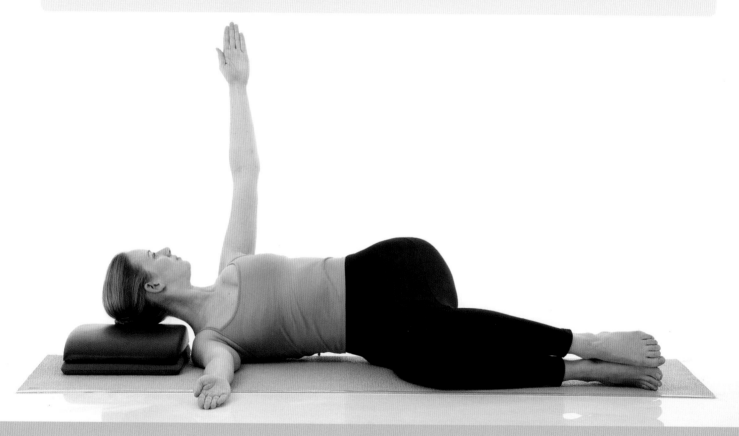

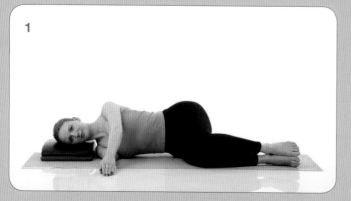

1

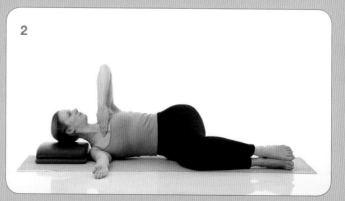

2

starting position

Lie on your right side and correctly align your pelvis and spine in neutral.

Place a substantial cushion underneath the head to ensure that your head and neck are in line with your spine. Bend both knees in front of you so that your hips and knees are bent to a right angle. Lengthen both arms out in front of your body at shoulder height. Your right arm is resting on the mat and your left arm is placed on top of the right.

Maintain an appropriate level of connection to your centre throughout.

action

● Breathe in as you bend your left elbow and slide your hand along the inside of the right arm to the centre of your breastbone. Simultaneously rotate your head, neck and upper spine but keep your pelvis and spine still.

● Breathe out as you rotate your spine further to the left. Encourage your breastbone and ribcage to soften.

● Breathe in and straighten your left elbow, lengthening your forearm away from your body. Maintain stillness and stability in your torso.

● Breathe out as you rotate and return your spine. Keep your left arm straight and move from the shoulder joint to return to the Starting Position.

Repeat up to five times, and then repeat on the other side.

WATCH POINTS

★ Ensure correct alignment in your side-lying starting position: shoulder above shoulder, hip above hip, knee above knee and foot above foot.

★ Ensure that your pelvis remains stable throughout.

★ Allow maximum rotation of the head and neck, but ensure length throughout.

★ Do not allow your arms to initiate the movement or move beyond the rotation of the spine.

★ Fully lengthen your arms but avoid locking your elbows.

★ The movement is ideally pure rotation. Continue to lengthen the spine, and avoid arching in your back or shortening in your waist.

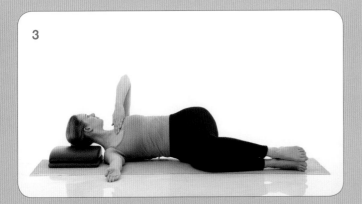

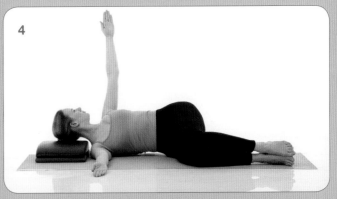

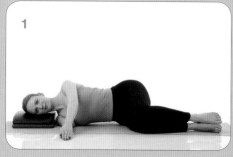

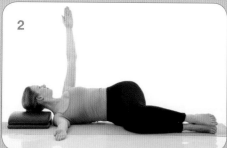

arm openings

Mobilise the head, neck and torso and promote openness and control around the shoulders.

starting position

Lie on your right side and correctly align your pelvis and spine in neutral. Place a substantial cushion underneath the head to ensure that your head and neck are in line with your spine. Bend both knees in front of you so that your hips and knees are bent to a right angle. Lengthen both arms out in front of your body at shoulder height. Your right arm is resting on the mat and your left arm is placed on top of the right.

Maintain an appropriate level of connection to your centre throughout.

action

● Breathe in as you raise the top arm, keeping it straight and lifting it above the shoulder joint towards the ceiling; simultaneously roll your head and neck to face the ceiling.

● Breathe out as you continue to rotate your head, neck and upper spine to the left, carry your left arm with your spine and open it further towards the mat. Your knees and pelvis remain still.

● Breathe in as you rotate your spine back to the right, initiating the movement from your centre. Simultaneously reach your left arm once again above the shoulder joint and towards the ceiling.

● Breathe out as you rotate and return your spine and arm back to the Starting Position.

Repeat up to five times, and then repeat on the other side.

WATCH POINTS

★ Ensure correct alignment in your side-lying starting position: shoulder above shoulder, hip above hip, knee above knee and foot above foot.

★ Ensure that your pelvis remains stable throughout.

★ The movement is ideally pure rotation. Continue to lengthen the spine, and avoid arching in your back or shortening in your waist.

★ Allow maximum rotation of the head and neck, but ensure length throughout.

★ Do not allow your arms to initiate the movement or move beyond the rotation of the spine.

tennis ball rising

Connects your body with your legs while mobilising and strengthening the ankles and feet.

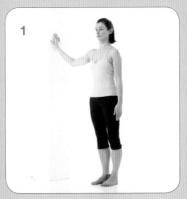

starting position

Stand tall on the floor (not on your mat) and lengthen your spine into neutral. Your legs are in parallel and slightly closer than hip-width apart; place a tennis ball in between your ankles, just below the inside ankle bones.

If necessary, stand sideways on to a wall and place your hand on the wall slightly in front of your body to help maintain balance.

Maintain an appropriate level of connection to your centre throughout.

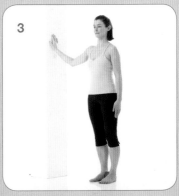

action

● Breathe in, preparing your body to move, and lengthen your spine.
● Breathe out and rise up onto the balls of your feet, lifting your heels off the floor. Keep your spine lengthened and stable and maintain the position of the ball in between your ankles.
● Breathe in. With control and maintaining length, lower your heels back down to the floor.
● Breathe out as you bend your knees, keeping your heels firmly on the floor.
● Breathe in as you straighten your legs and return to the Starting Position. Repeat up to ten times.

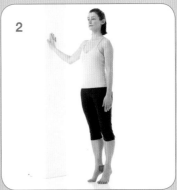

WATCH POINTS

★ Maintain a neutral pelvis and spine throughout. Remain long in your waist and keep a sense of your spine lengthening up and away.

★ Fully lengthen your legs but avoid locking your knees.

★ Keep your weight balanced evenly on both feet. Also, do not allow your feet to roll either in or out.

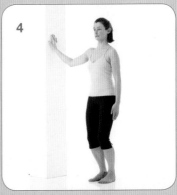

single leg stretch – preparation

Develops the coordination and strength needed to perform the full exercise. Strengthens the abdominals and mobilises the hips and knees.

starting position

It may be a good idea to wear socks for this exercise to enable your feet to slide freely along the mat/floor.

Align yourself correctly in the Relaxation Position. Double Knee Fold one leg at a time with stability; connect your inner thighs and softly point your feet.

Breathe in, preparing your body to move and, as you breathe out, nod your head and sequentially wheel your neck and upper body off the mat into a Curl Up position. Lengthen your arms forwards and place your hands on the outside of your shins.

Maintain an appropriate level of connection to your centre throughout.

action

● Breathe into the back of your ribcage as you hold the curled-up position.

● Breathe out as you lower your right leg to the mat. Keep your knee bent and touch your toes to the mat first, simultaneously placing the right hand on the left knee. Once your foot is placed on the mat, slide your leg along the mat, straightening it out in line with your hip as you gently draw the left leg in towards your torso.

● Breathe in and, maintaining your curled-up position, slide your right leg back in towards your body. Once the knee is bent sufficiently, fold your leg up and in. Return your right hand to your left shinbone.

Repeat on the other leg. Focus on sliding your straight leg away from your body as you gently draw the bent leg in towards you.

Repeat the whole sequence up to five times.

To finish, remain curled up and bend both knees in towards your torso. Roll your upper spine and head back down to the mat and then, maintaining a stable pelvis, return your feet to the mat to finish in the Relaxation Position.

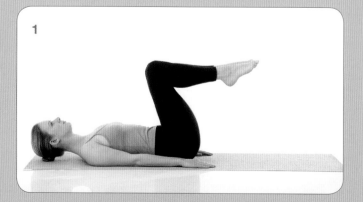

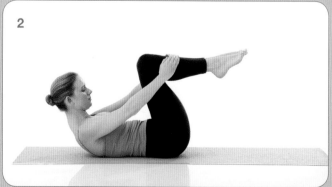

WATCH POINTS

★ Ensure that your pelvis remains grounded in neutral throughout; curl up only as far as this can be maintained.

★ Focus on moving your legs independently from your pelvis and spine.

★ As you lengthen the leg away from you, focus on fully straightening the leg but avoid locking your knee.

★ Maintain the curled-up position. Use your arms to draw your legs towards you and not to pull your spine up further.

★ Maintain length in your neck, and keep your head still. Focus down onto your abdominal area.

★ Allow your collarbones to widen, but keep a connection of the shoulder blades to the back of the ribcage.

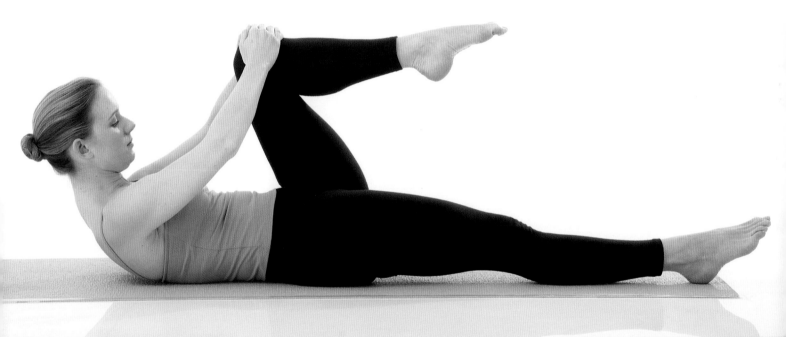

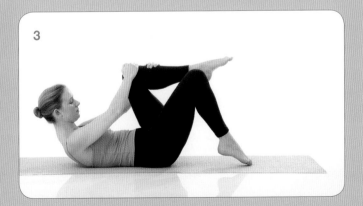

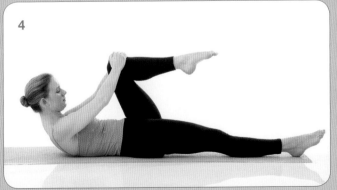

WATCH POINTS

★ Ensure that your pelvis remains grounded in neutral throughout; move your arms and legs independently from your pelvis and spine.

★ Both your arms and legs should move at the same time, creating opposition, length and openness across the front of your body.

★ Ensure that you maintain the curled-up position of the spine throughout. It is very easy to lose this flexion as the arms and legs reach away.

★ Maintain length in your neck, and keep your head still; focus down onto your abdominal area.

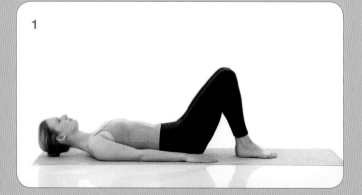

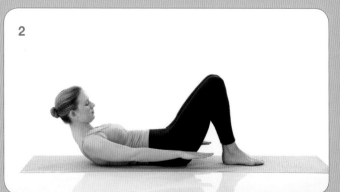

double leg stretch – preparation

Challenges core stability, strengthens the abdominals and mobilises the hip, knee and shoulder joints while developing coordination.

starting position

It may be a good idea to wear socks for this exercise to enable your feet to slide freely along the mat/floor.

Align yourself correctly in the Relaxation Position, lengthening your arms by the side of your body on the mat. Bring your legs together and connect your inner thighs.

Breathe in, preparing your body to move and, as you breathe out, nod your head and sequentially wheel your neck and upper body off the mat into a Curl Up position. Raise your arms slightly off the mat and lengthen them forwards.

Maintain an appropriate level of connection to your centre throughout.

action

● Breathe in, remain curled up and straighten both legs, sliding them along the mat. Simultaneously reach your straight arms overhead, shoulder-width apart.

● Breathe out as you bend your knees and slide your feet along the mat, bringing your legs back in towards you. Simultaneously circle the arms out to the side and around, to return to their lengthened position alongside your torso. Remain curled up throughout.

Repeat up to ten times.

To finish, roll your upper spine and head back down to the mat.

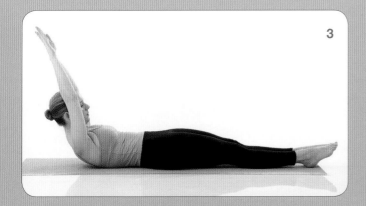
3

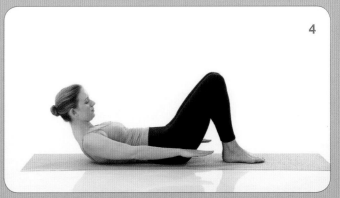
4

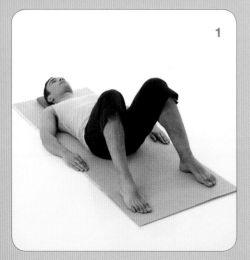

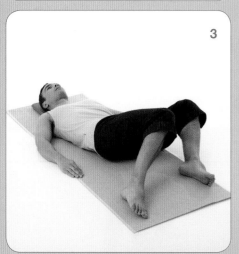

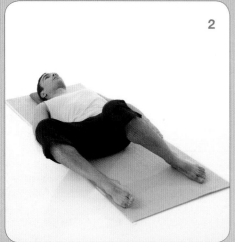

knee rolls

Help to increase mobility in the hip joints while trying to maintain a stable relationship between the hip, knee and ankle joints.

starting position

Align yourself correctly in the Relaxation Position. Position your legs slightly wider than hip-width apart. Reach your arms out on the mat slightly lower than shoulder height with your palms facing down.

Maintain an appropriate level of connection to your centre throughout.

action

- Breathe in, preparing your body to move.
- Breathe out as you roll your left leg in from the hip joint and simultaneously roll the right leg out, also from the hip joint. Both knees will therefore roll to the right; allow your feet to peel slightly off the mat.
- Breathe out and return both legs back to the centre at the same time.

Repeat to the other side and then repeat the whole sequence up to five times.

WATCH POINTS

★ Unlike Hip Rolls, the initiation for this action should come from the legs, specifically the top of your thigh in the hip socket.

★ Attempt to keep your pelvis still and square; although there will be slight reactionary movement, it is not your main objective to rotate the pelvis and spine.

★ Although you should have a sense of release in your hip joints, control the movement of your legs and don't just allow them to 'drop' to the side.

oyster

Helps to mobilise your hips while strengthening the muscles around the joint.

starting position

Lie on your right side, in a straight line, correctly stacking your shoulders, hips and ankles. Your pelvis and spine should remain in neutral. Lengthen your right arm underneath your head and in line with your spine. Place your left hand on the mat in front of your ribcage and bend your elbow to support your position lightly. Bend both knees in front of you and draw your feet back so that your heels are aligned with the back of your pelvis.

Maintain an appropriate level of connection to your centre throughout.

action

- Breathe in, preparing your body to move.
- Breathe out and, maintaining a neutral pelvis and spine, open your top knee, keeping your feet connected together. This 'turn-out' movement will come from your hip joint.
- Breathe in and with control return your leg to the Starting Position.

Repeat up to ten times and then repeat on the other side.

WATCH POINTS

★ Ensure correct alignment in your side-lying starting position: shoulder above shoulder, hip above hip and knee above knee.

★ Ensure that your pelvis remains stable throughout. The action of the leg opening must come from your hip joint: your leg moves in isolation from the rest your body.

★ Open your top leg only as far as you can without disturbing the position of your pelvis.

★ Keep lengthening both sides of the waist throughout.

★ The top arm is positioned to help support you, but avoid placing too much weight onto it.

★ Keep your chest open, and your focus directly ahead of you.

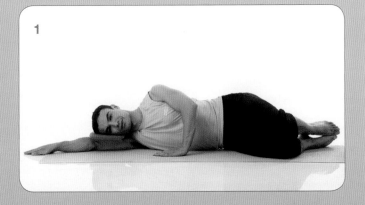

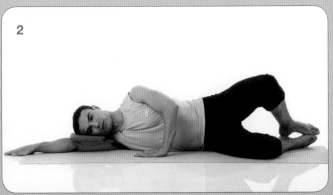

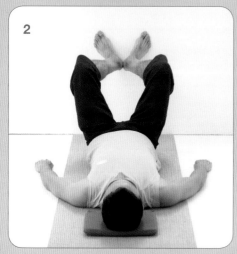

1

2

3

zigzags – lying

Improve and maintain mobility in the hip joints.

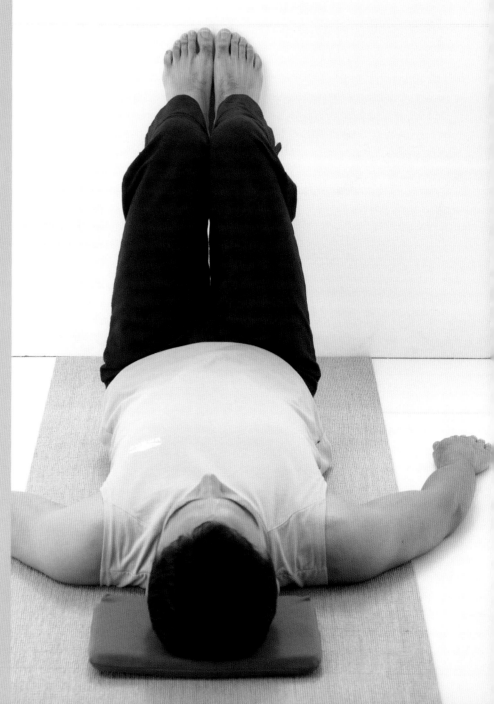

starting position

Align yourself correctly in the Relaxation Position and place your feet up onto a wall. Ideally your thighs will be vertical and your shins will be horizontal; your pelvis and spine remain in neutral. Bring your legs together and connect your inner thighs; the soles of your feet are flat against the wall.
Maintain an appropriate level of connection to your centre throughout.

action

- Breathe in as you turn your legs out slightly from your hips, opening your knees and sliding your feet to a small 'V' position; keep the heels together.
- Breathe out as you turn the legs in, again moving from your hip joints and drawing your knees naturally towards one another; your heels will slide away from one another.
- Continue to 'zigzag' your legs and feet up to six times until the legs are at a comfortable distance apart.
- Reverse the movement and, in the same amount of repetitions, 'zigzag' the legs back to the Starting Position.
Repeat up to ten times.

WATCH POINTS

★ Keep your pelvis and spine stable and still throughout; focus on the independent movement of the thigh bone in the hip socket.

★ Although you should have a sense of release in your hip joints, control the movement of your legs and don't just allow them to 'drop' to the side.

★ Maintain correct alignment of the legs; your feet, knees and hips should remain correctly aligned and move together. It is very easy to press your feet or your knees out further than your hips can turn out, but is essential that this be avoided.

★ Avoid lifting your feet off the wall; allow the soles of your feet to slide.

★ Keep your chest and the front of your shoulders open and avoid any tension in your neck area.

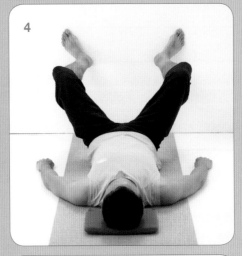

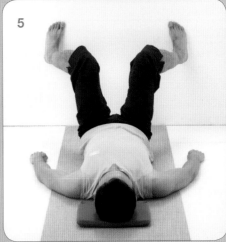

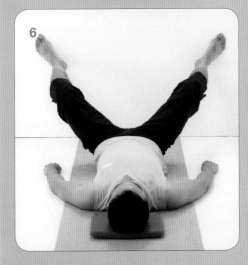

73

zigzags – sitting

This is a great exercise for increasing mobility in the hip joints while trying to maintain a stable relationship between the hip, knee and ankle joints. It also challenges the stability of your spine as the legs move independently from the hips.

starting position

Sit upright with your legs lengthened out in front of your body. Straighten your arms and circle them behind your body, to place the palms on the mat for support. Place your legs slightly wider than hip-width apart, turn them out from the hips, flex your feet and bend your knees to draw the legs in towards you as far as is possible whilst still maintaining a neutral pelvis and spine. Maintain an appropriate level of connection to your centre throughout.

action

● Breathe in, preparing your body to move, and lengthen your spine.
● Breathe out and, maintaining length and stability in your spine, straighten your legs, sliding your feet along the mat while maintaining the turned-out position and the flexed feet.
● Breathe in. Keeping your legs straight, roll your legs in from the hips.
● Breathe out and, maintaining the turned-in position of your legs, bend your knees and draw your legs back in towards your body, sliding the feet along the mat.
● Breathe in. Keeping your legs bent, turn your legs out from the hips, returning to the Starting Position.
Repeat up to five times and then reverse the direction.

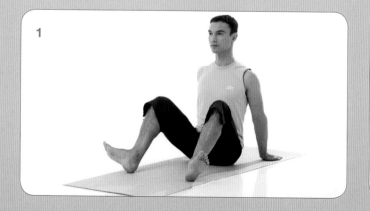

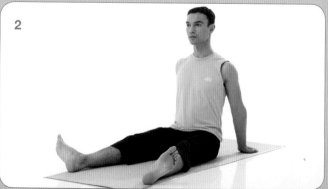

WATCH POINTS

★ Keep your pelvis and spine stable and still throughout; focus on the independent movement of the thigh bone in the hip socket.

★ Although you should have a sense of release in your hip joints, control the movement of your legs and don't just allow them to 'drop' to the side.

★ Maintain correct alignment of the legs; your feet, knees and hips should remain correctly aligned and move together. It is really easy to press your feet or your knees out further than your hips can turn out, but is essential that this be avoided.

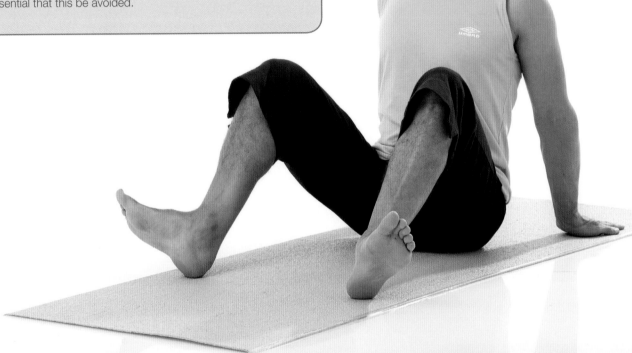

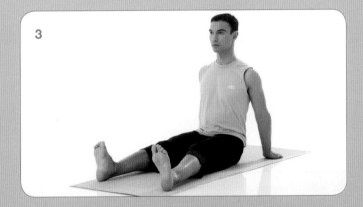

3

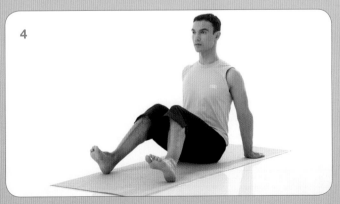

4

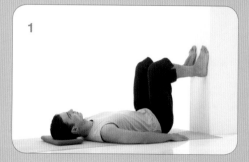

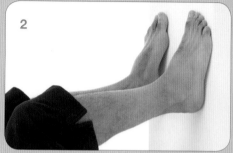

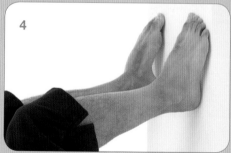

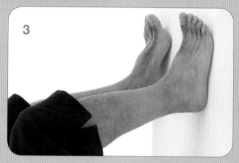

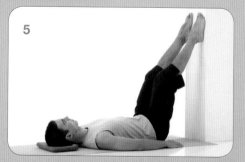

creeping feet

Mobilises the feet and ankles and helps develop support around your arches.

starting position

Align yourself correctly in the Relaxation Position and place your feet up onto a wall. Ideally your thighs will be vertical and your shins will be horizontal; your pelvis and spine remain in neutral. Place your legs hip-width apart and parallel, the soles of your feet are flat against the wall.

This exercise can also be performed sitting upright on a chair, with your feet hip-width apart on the floor.

Maintain an appropriate level of connection to your centre throughout.

action

Breathe naturally throughout.

● Pick up your toes and spread your feet and toes as wide as possible onto the wall, and then lift up the arches of the feet and glide the heels up the wall. Maintain contact of the feet to the wall throughout.

● Repeat as above and continue creeping your feet up the wall until they can no longer stay flat.

● Bend your knees and slide your feet back down the wall, returning to the Starting Position.

Repeat up to ten times.

WATCH POINTS

★ Avoid over-curling the toes and creating tension; try to keep the action in the arches of the feet.

★ Ensure that your feet remain evenly grounded and aligned on the wall and do not roll out or in.

★ Maintain correct alignment of your hips, knees and ankles.

mexican wave

Mobilises the joints of the foot and teaches you how to coordinate and control the feet.

starting position

Stand tall on the floor (not on your mat) and lengthen your spine into neutral. Your legs are in parallel and hip-width apart. Allow your arms to lengthen down by the sides of your body.

This exercise can also be performed sitting upright on a chair, with your feet grounded hip-width apart on the floor.

Maintain an appropriate level of connection to your centre throughout.

action

Breathe naturally throughout.

● First, lift only your big toes off the floor, keeping the rest of your toes down. Then, try to lift your toes one at a time in sequence until all of the toes have peeled off the floor.

● Replace your toes back down in sequence, starting with the little toe and spacing them out as wide as possible.

● Reverse the movement: raise the little toes first, continuing one toe at a time to the big toe.

Repeat up to five times, either working the feet separately or both together.

WATCH POINTS

★　Maintain correct alignment of your leg: ensure that your foot, ankle and knee remain in line with your hip.

★　Continue to maintain a stable and lengthened vertical position of your pelvis and spine throughout.

★　Keep your chest and the front of your shoulders open and avoid any tension in your neck area.

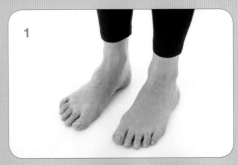

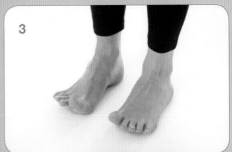

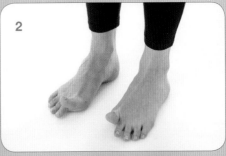

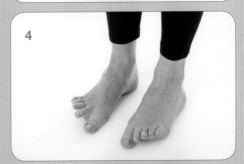

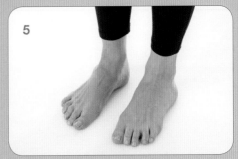

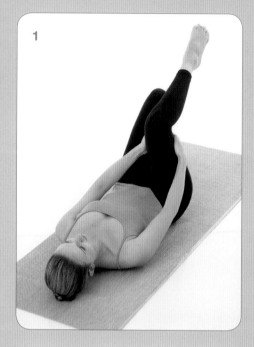

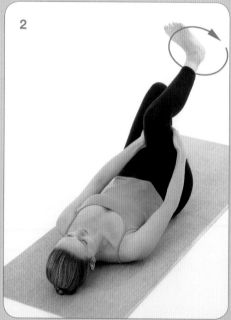

ankle circles

Help to mobilise the ankle joints and release tension around the lower leg.

starting position

Align yourself correctly in the Relaxation Position. Fold one leg in towards your body with stability. Clasp your hands lightly behind your thigh and lift your lower leg up slightly so that your foot is higher than your knee.

This exercise can also be performed sitting upright on the mat with your legs lengthened out in front of you and your arms reaching behind your body with your hands resting on the mat for support.

Maintain an appropriate level of connection to your centre throughout.

action

Breathe naturally throughout.

● Keeping your leg still, flex your foot, moving only your ankle joint, and circle your foot outwards. Complete a full circle, trying to keep your foot and toes lengthened and free from tension.

● Repeat the ankle circle up to five times and then reverse the direction and circle the ankle up to five times inwards.

Repeat on the other ankle, up to five times in each direction.

WATCH POINTS

★ Maintain a neutral pelvis and spine throughout. Particularly avoid twisting your pelvis or side-bending your spine as you reach to hold your leg.

★ Keep your thigh and shins still and correctly aligned throughout. Remember, you want the circle to come purely from your ankle.

★ Try to keep your toes from being 'over-active'. For a foot and toe workout, try Mexican Wave (page 77) or Creeping Feet (page 76).

standing on one leg

Centres the body, while strengthening the ankles and feet by challenging your balance.

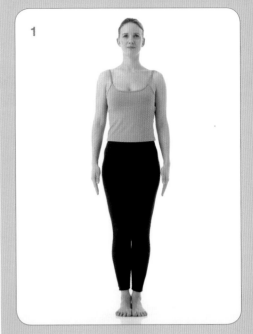

starting position

Stand tall on the floor (not on your mat) and lengthen your spine into neutral. Bring your legs together and connect your inner thighs in parallel.
Maintain an appropriate level of connection to your centre throughout.

action

● Breathe in, preparing your body to move, and lengthen your spine.
● Breathe out, transfer your weight onto your left leg and, keeping the pelvis as level as possible, bend your right knee to lift your foot slightly off the floor and draw your leg up and in towards your torso.
● Breathe in as you hold this lengthened and stable position, feeling the opposition of the crown of your head reaching away from your grounded left foot.
● Breathe out, return your right leg back to the standing position and evenly distribute your weight through both feet.
Repeat up to five times on each side, alternating legs.

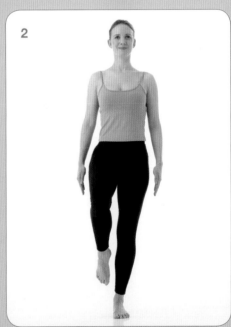

WATCH POINTS

★ Maintain a neutral pelvis and spine throughout. Lengthen both sides of the waist and avoid 'hitching' your pelvis up towards your ribcage.

★ Fully lengthen your supporting leg but avoid locking the knee.

★ Maintain the parallel alignment of your supporting leg; ensure that your knee remains facing forwards.

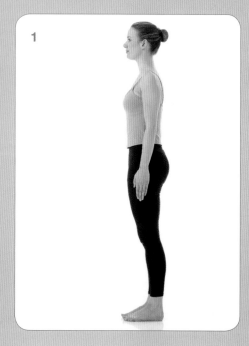

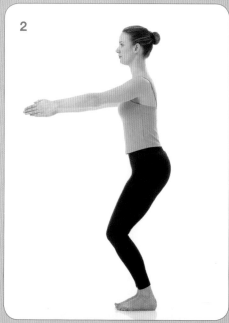

pilates squats

Strengthen and balance the leg muscles; also mobilise and coordinate the hip, knee and ankle joints while challenging spinal stability.

starting position

Stand tall on the floor (not on your mat) and lengthen your spine into neutral. Your legs are in parallel and hip-width apart. Allow your arms to lengthen down by the sides of your body, palms facing inwards.

Maintain an appropriate level of connection to your centre throughout.

action

● Breathe in, lengthen your spine and bend your knees, feeling the deep crease in the front of your hips. Maintaining neutral alignment, naturally allow your torso to tilt forwards slightly and simultaneously allow your arms to lengthen and rise up to shoulder height.

● Breathe out and, grounding your feet down into the floor, straighten your legs and return your spine to the upright Starting Position. Simultaneously lower the arms back down by your sides.

Repeat up to ten times.

WATCH POINTS

★ Maintain a neutral pelvis and spine throughout. The pitching forwards of the spine is a natural counterbalance to the bending of the knees and occurs through the hinging of your hips.

★ Remain long in your waist and keep a sense of your spine lengthening up and away.

★ Keep your weight balanced evenly on both feet and do not allow them to roll in or out.

wrist circles

Mobilise the wrist joints and are a good way to release tension around the forearm.

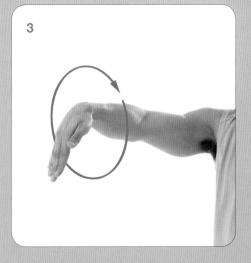

starting position

Stand tall on the floor (not on your mat) and lengthen your spine into neutral. Your legs are either parallel and hip-width apart or connected in Pilates Stance. Allow your arms to lengthen down by the sides of your body.

Lengthening through your fingertips, raise your arms forwards and up to shoulder height, and then slightly bend your elbows, keeping your palms facing down. Maintain an appropriate level of connection to your centre throughout.

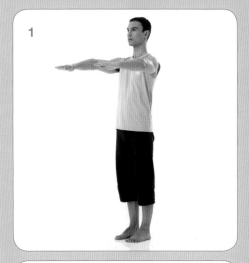

action

Breathe naturally throughout.

● Keeping your shoulders relaxed and your upper arms still, begin to circle both your wrists inwards and around, completing a full, even circle. Keep the hands and fingers lengthened and free from tension.

Repeat the wrist circle five times and then reverse the direction and circle the wrists five times outwards.

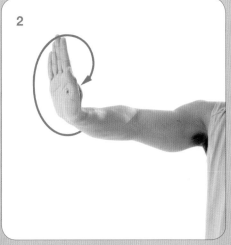

WATCH POINTS

★ Keep your hands open and lengthened throughout; the movement comes from the wrist joint and does not involve the fingers.

★ Although it is necessary to keep your upper arms still, you will notice a certain amount of rotation in your forearms.

★ Remain lengthened in your neck, open in the chest and relaxed in your shoulders. If you do feel any tension, lower your arms slightly.

★ Attempt to create full and even circles.

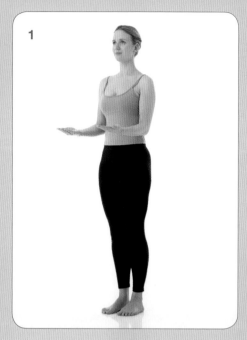

dumb waiter

Re-balances the movement of the upper arm in relation to the shoulder blades, promoting openness across the front of the shoulders.

starting position

Stand tall on the floor (not on your mat) and lengthen your spine into neutral. Your legs are in parallel and hip-width apart. Bend your elbows to an approximate right angle; your upper arm is positioned vertically, and your forearm is lengthening forwards horizontally. Turn your palms to face upwards.

This exercise can also be performed sitting upright on a chair, with your feet grounded hip-width apart on the floor.

Maintain an appropriate level of connection to your centre throughout.

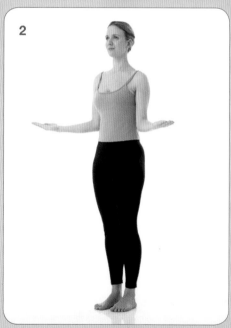

action

● Breathe in and, keeping your elbows directly underneath your shoulders, turn your arms outwards from the shoulder joint, reaching your forearms wide.
● Breathe out as you return the arms back to the Starting Position; your forearms are once again parallel.

Repeat up to ten times.

WATCH POINTS

★ Continue to maintain a stable and lengthened vertical position of your pelvis and spine throughout.

★ Ensure that the movement comes from the shoulder joint alone. Do not squeeze your shoulder blades together, but instead focus on them remaining wide across the back of your ribcage.

★ Keep your chest and the front of your shoulders open. Release your neck and lengthen your head upwards.

roll downs – against a wall

Help to mobilise the spine and hips, strengthening the muscles of your back, buttocks and legs.

starting position

Stand tall with your back against a wall. Place your feet in parallel and hip-width apart, approximately 30cm from the wall, and bend your knees slightly. Your pelvis is in neutral and should feel supported by the wall. Your spine is also in neutral, so you will feel its natural curves. The back of the head may or may not be in contact depending on your individual posture. Allow your arms to lengthen down by the sides.

action

- Breathe in as you lengthen the back of your neck and nod your head forwards.
- Breathe out as you roll your entire spine forwards and down. First soften your breastbone and then wheel your lower ribcage before gently imprinting your lower spine into the wall. Roll until you can go no further without your hips hinging.
- Breathe in as you begin to roll your pelvis underneath you.
- Breathe out as you continue to roll your spine back up, replacing each vertebra against the wall. Lengthen your spine as you return back to neutral.
Repeat up to ten times.

WATCH POINTS

★ Roll smoothly and sequentially through each segment of your spine.

★ Roll directly through your centre line, avoiding any deviations to either side.

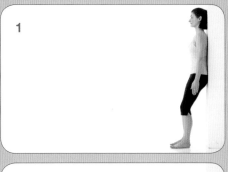

1

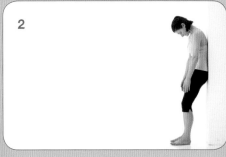

2

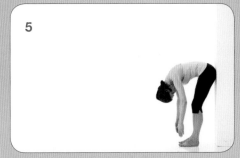

3

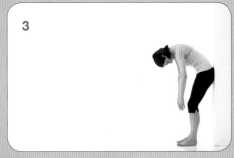

4

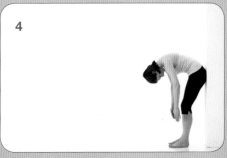

5

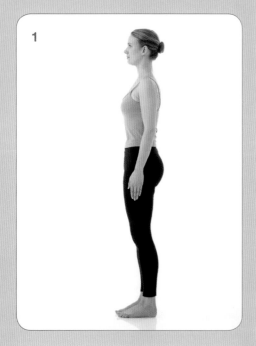

1

roll downs – freestanding

Once you have got the hang of Roll Downs – against a wall, try this exercise freestanding. Without the feedback and support of the wall it is essential to maintain awareness of your movement and a strong connection to your centre throughout.

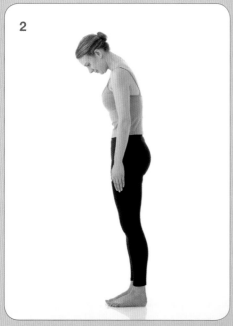

2

starting position

Stand tall on the floor (not on your mat) and lengthen your spine into neutral. Your legs are in parallel and hip-width apart. Allow your arms to lengthen down by the sides of your body.

Maintain an appropriate level of connection to your centre throughout.

action

● Breathe in as you lengthen the back of your neck and nod your head forwards.
● Breathe out as you continue to roll your entire spine forwards and down. Firstly soften your breastbone and then wheel your ribcage forward before allowing your lower back to curl and open. Roll until you can go no further without your hips hinging.
● Breathe in as you begin to roll your pelvis underneath you.
● Breathe out as you continue to roll your spine back up, restacking each vertebra one at a time. Lengthen your spine as you return back to neutral.
Repeat up to ten times.

WATCH POINTS

★ Remember to connect your abdominals to support your spine.

★ Keep your weight balanced evenly on both feet. Also, do not allow your feet to roll either in or out.

★ Focus on the control of the movement with your breath and keep the whole movement even-paced and flowing.

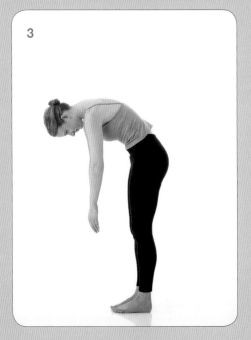

3

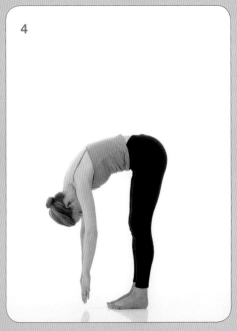

4

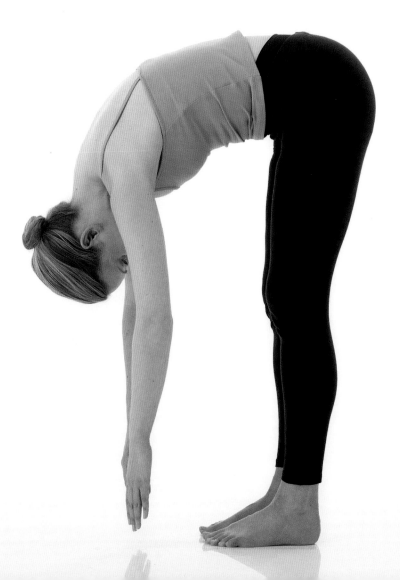

workouts

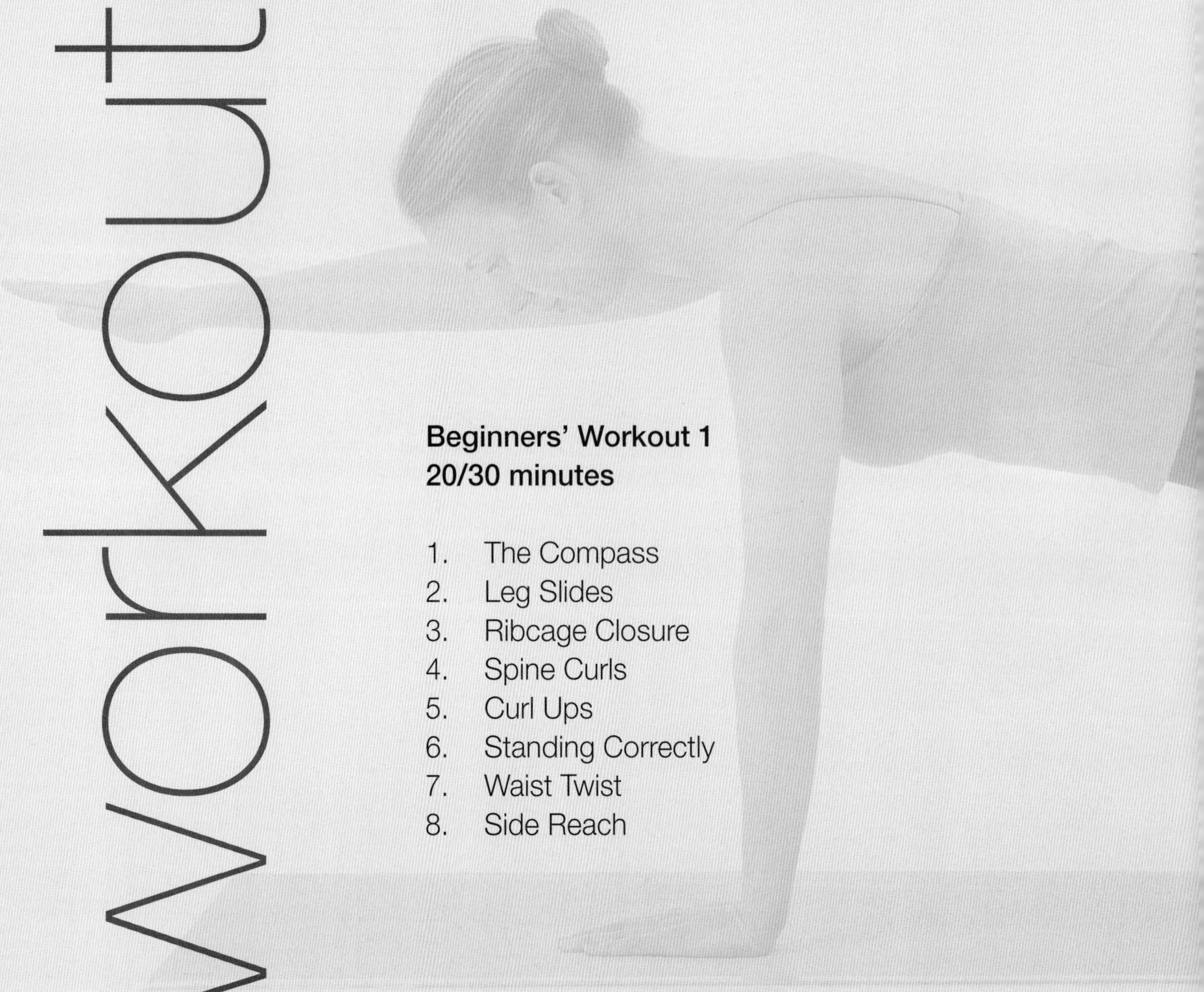

**Beginners' Workout 1
20/30 minutes**

1. The Compass
2. Leg Slides
3. Ribcage Closure
4. Spine Curls
5. Curl Ups
6. Standing Correctly
7. Waist Twist
8. Side Reach

Beginners' Workout 2
40/50 minutes

1. Shoulder Drops
2. Knee Openings
3. Single Knee Folds
4. Spine Curls
5. Arm Circles
6. Curl Ups
7. Hip Rolls – Feet Down
8. Table Top
9. The Cat
10. Diamond Press
11. Rest Position
12. Bow and Arrow – Sitting
13. Side Reach – Sitting
14. Oyster
15. Tennis Ball Rising
16. Roll Downs – Against a Wall

Beginners' Workout 3
60/70 minutes

1. Pelvic Clocks
2. Windows
3. Knee Circles
4. Curl Ups
5. Single Leg Stretch – Preparation
6. Spine Curls
7. Double Knee Fold
8. Hip Rolls – Feet Up
9. Double Leg Stretch – Preparation
10. Zigzags – Sitting
11. Bow and Arrow – Sitting
12. Dart
13. Cobra Prep
14. Rest Position
15. The Cat
16. Oyster
17. Arm Openings
18. Pilates Stance
19. Dumb Waiter
20. Pilates Squats
21. Floating Arms
22. Side Reach – Standing
23. Roll Downs – Freestanding

Chapter Three:
The Intermediate
Matwork Programme

In this section we have introduced some new exercises to challenge you further, once you have mastered the beginners' exercises. This selection includes many Classical Pilates exercises that go to make up the Advanced Matwork Sequence (page 166). Admittedly some of these exercises are very difficult, so take your time, be patient and continue to refer back to the fundamental and beginners' exercises to help you to build your strength and understand the technique.

Once again, to help you to group together a balanced selection of exercises, we have suggested Intermediate Workouts for you of different lengths (page 130).

the exercises

1. The Hundred
2. Roll Backs
3. Roll Up
4. Roll Over
5. Leg Circles
6. Rolling Like a Ball
7. Single Leg Stretch
8. Double Leg Stretch
9. Single Straight Leg Stretch
10. Double Straight Leg Raises
11. Criss-cross
12. Spine Stretch Forward
13. Open Leg Rocker
14. The Saw

15. Cobra
16. Single Leg Kick
17. Double Leg Kick
18. Spine Twist
19. Side Kick Series – Front and Back
20. Side Kick Series – Up and Down
21. Side Kick Series – Small Circles
22. Prone Beats
23. Torpedo
24. Leg Pull Front
25. Leg Pull Back
26. Star
27. Seal
28. Mermaid

the hundred

Challenges the endurance of the abdominal, hip and leg muscles and releases unwanted tension in the upper body.

starting position

Align yourself correctly in the Relaxation Position. Double Knee Fold one leg at a time with stability, keeping your heels connected and your feet softly pointed, knees slightly open. (If performing the Advanced Matwork Sequence, connect your inner thighs and lift both legs off the mat at the same time.)

Breathe in, preparing your body to move, and as you breathe out, nod your head and sequentially wheel your neck and upper body off the mat into a Curl Up position. Simultaneously straighten and slightly lower your legs, connecting the inner thighs in Pilates Stance. Maintaining the length in the arms, raise them slightly from the mat.

Maintain an appropriate level of connection to your centre throughout.

action

● Breathe in for a count of five and, remaining curled up, beat the arms up and down five times.

● Breathe out for a count of five, focus on a full exhalation, and again beat the arms up and down five times.

Repeat ten times to one hundred.

To finish, remain curled up as you bend the knees in towards your torso. Roll your upper spine and head back down to the mat and then, maintaining a stable pelvis, return your feet to the mat to finish in the Relaxation Position. (If performing the Advanced Matwork Sequence, connect your inner thighs and return both legs to the mat at the same time.)

Variation

If you find maintaining the position of your legs difficult, try bending your knees so your legs remain lifted. If this is still too challenging, you could leave your feet on the mat.

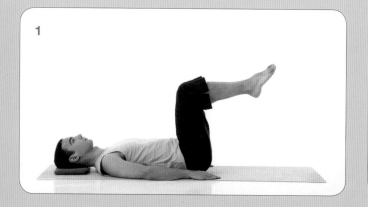

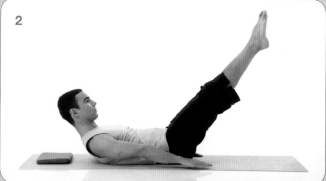

WATCH POINTS

★ Ensure that your pelvis remains grounded in neutral throughout. Lower your legs only to a point where this can still be maintained.

★ Focus on the ribs gently expanding on the inhalation and drawing together on the exhalation.

★ Allow your collarbones and shoulder blades to widen, but keep a connection of the shoulder blades to the back of the ribcage.

★ Maintain length in your neck, and keep your head still. Focus down onto your abdominal area.

★ Keep your arms straight and lengthened but be careful not to lock your elbows.

★ Ensure the movement of the arms comes purely from the shoulders.

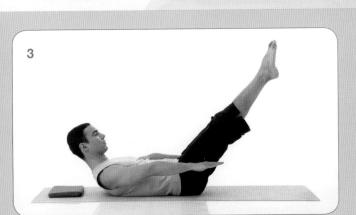

3

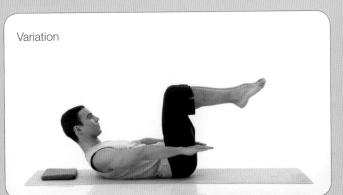

Variation

roll backs

Prepare your body for the Roll Up by strengthening the abdominals and hips while challenging the C-Curved alignment of the spine.

starting position

Sit upright with your knees bent and the soles of your feet grounded on the mat. Your legs are hip-width apart and your pelvis and spine are in neutral. Reach your arms out in front of you, slightly lower than shoulder height and shoulder-width apart. Your arms are lengthened, and your palms are facing down. Maintain an appropriate level of connection to your centre throughout.

action

● Breathe in as you lengthen the spine into a C-Curve, shoulders over the hips.
● Breathe out, as you roll the pelvis and your flexed spine backwards, until the back of your pelvis is supported by the mat.
● Breathe in as you maintain your roll-back position, ensuring the spine is still in a C-Curve.
● Breathe out as you initiate with your head and roll the C-Curved spine forwards, returning your shoulders over your hips. Then, moving the pelvis and head simultaneously, lengthen your spine back to neutral.
Repeat up to ten times.

Variation

Place your hands behind the thighs. As your spine rolls backwards, allow your hands to slide along the back of the thighs towards the pelvis, and, as your spine rolls forwards, allow them to slide back towards your knees. Your arms must be used to guide and control the movement, not to pull your body up.

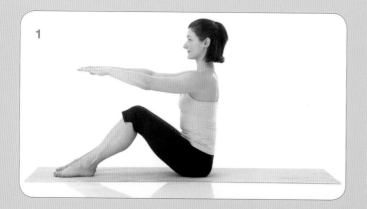

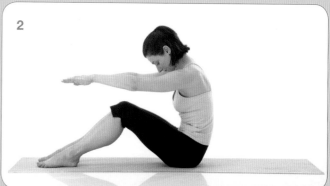

WATCH POINTS

★ Maintain a curved (flexed) spine throughout. Once the C-Curve has been established, it is merely the pelvis rolling away from the legs that creates the movement; the C-Curve is maintained.

★ The C-Curve is a lengthened position; avoid any compression and feel support from the abdominals.

★ Encourage an equal amount of flexion throughout the entire length of your spine.

★ Roll directly through your centreline, avoiding any deviations.

★ Maintain openness across your chest and the back of your shoulders, avoiding over-reaching forwards with your arms and allow the arms to move naturally with the spine as it rolls backwards.

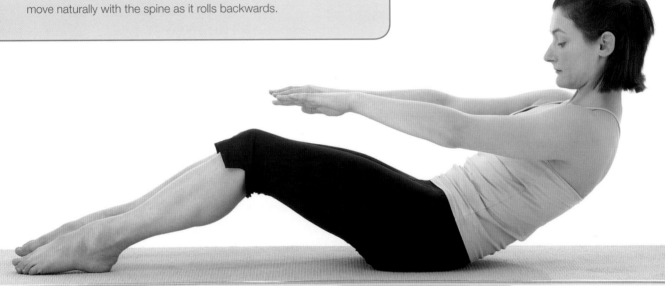

3

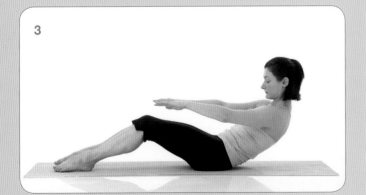

Variation:

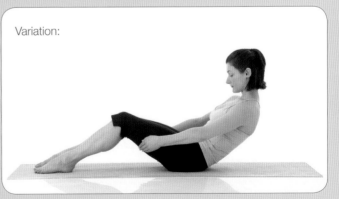

roll up

starting position

Lie on your back with both legs straight and connected together in parallel with your feet flexed. Your pelvis and spine are in neutral. Raise your arms overhead with your palms facing up and maintain openness across the chest.

Maintain an appropriate level of connection to your centre throughout.

action

● Breathe in as you raise your arms and simultaneously begin to roll up from your head, neck and upper back.

● Breathe out as you continue to roll the rest of the spine, sequentially wheeling it off the mat, one vertebra at a time. Lengthen the C-Curved spine over your legs. Reach the arms forward, ensuring they maintain their relationship with your neck and head.

● Breathe in as you begin to roll the pelvis and spine back along the mat, ensuring that you initiate the movement from the pelvis.

● Breathe out as you continue to wheel the whole spine sequentially down onto the mat, returning the head and the arms on the final part of your exhalation.

Repeat up to ten times.

WATCH POINTS

★ Ensure that you roll smoothly through each segment of your spine. Do not roll forwards from your hips until the spine is fully flexed into a C-Curve.

★ Beware not to curl forwards excessively from the head and neck; remember that you are looking for a balanced C-Curve shape in the spine.

★ Maintain length throughout your spine; avoid any shortening or compression of the spine, particularly as you roll down.

★ Roll directly through your centre line, avoiding any deviations to either side.

★ Keep a relationship between the shoulders and the back of your ribcage. Neither force them to depress, nor allow them to over-elevate, especially while reaching forwards over the legs.

★ Focus on the control of the movement with your breath and keep the whole movement even-paced and flowing.

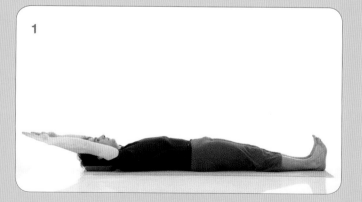

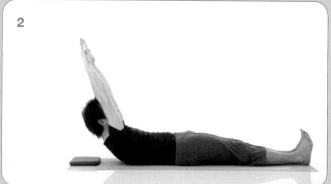

Promotes mobilisation of the spine and hips while challenging the balance of strength and mobility throughout the whole body.

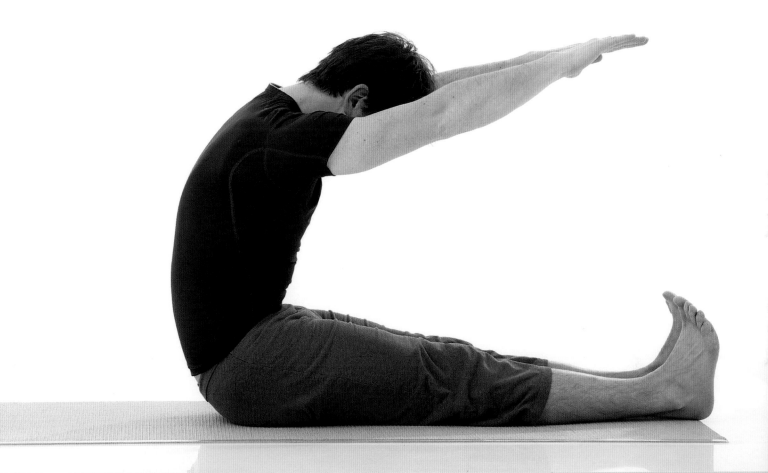

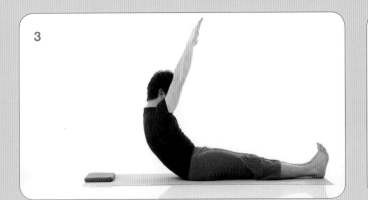

3

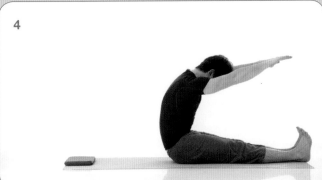

4

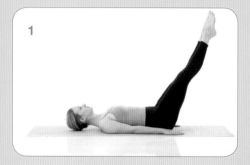

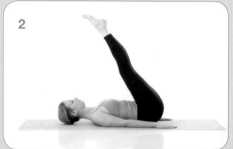

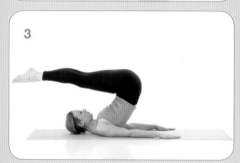

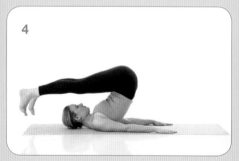

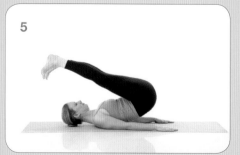

roll over

Helps develop strength along the front of the body and legs as well as the back of the arms.

starting position

Align yourself correctly in the Relaxation Position. Double Knee Fold one leg at a time with stability, connect your inner thighs and softly point your feet. Straighten both legs directly above your pelvis and then lower them to a point where you can still maintain a neutral pelvis and spine; do not allow your lower back to arch. (If performing the Advanced Matwork Sequence, connect your inner thighs and lift both legs off the mat at the same time.) Maintain an appropriate level of connection to your centre throughout. The movement is continuous, flowing and dynamic without momentum. The breathing pattern is essential to achieving this.

action

● Breathe in as you lengthen the legs and begin to draw them in towards your body; keep your pelvis down for as long as possible.
● Breathe out as you allow your pelvis and spine to roll sequentially off the mat, drawing the legs up and over your torso until they are parallel with the mat. Make

WATCH POINTS

★ Initiate the movement from a strong centre; avoid momentum.

★ Focus on maintaining length in the spine, avoiding any compression, especially as the legs lower in the Roll Over position.

★ Avoid rolling too far over. The weight should be across the upper back, not the head and neck. Maintain length in the neck.

★ Keep the chest open and the arms reaching along the mat, and if necessary press down with the upper arm to help initiation and control.

★ As you roll the spine, maintain correct alignment with your centre line.

sure that you do not roll too far; there should not be any pressure on the neck and head or tension in the shoulders.

● Breathe in as you open the legs to shoulder-width and flex your feet. Without deepening the curve of the spine attempt to lower both legs a little nearer the mat.

● Breathe out and, with control, sequentially roll the spine and pelvis back down along the mat. Keep the legs close to the front of the body until your pelvis and spine have returned to neutral.

● Still breathing out, lower the legs away from your torso, towards the mat as far as possible, without losing your neutral spinal alignment. Softly point your feet and connect your legs together.

Repeat three times. On the third repetition return the legs directly above the pelvis, keeping the legs apart and your feet flexed; repeat the Roll Over a further three times with the reverse leg pattern:

● Breathe in as you hinge the legs towards your body, keeping your pelvis down for as long as possible. (The legs are now shoulder-width apart and the feet flexed.)

● Breathe out as you allow your pelvis and spine to roll sequentially off the mat, drawing the legs up and over your torso until they are parallel with the mat.

● Breathe in as you close the legs and softly point your feet. Then, without deepening the curve of the spine, attempt to lower both legs a little nearer the mat.

● Breathe out and, with control, sequentially roll the spine and pelvis back down along the mat. Keep the legs close to the front of the body until your pelvis and spine have returned to neutral.

● Still breathing out, lower the legs away from the body towards the mat as far as possible, without losing your neutral spinal alignment; close the legs together and softly point your feet.

Repeat the reverse direction three times.

To finish, once you have completed three repetitions with reverse legs, return the legs directly above the pelvis, then bend the knees and, maintaining a stable pelvis, return your legs one at a time to the mat to end in the Relaxation Position.

(If performing the Advanced Matwork Sequence, connect your inner thighs and return both legs to the mat at the same time.)

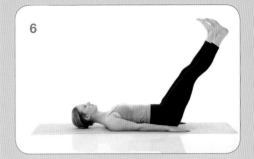

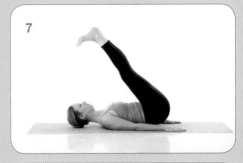

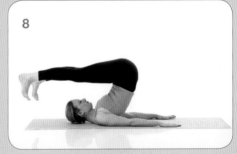

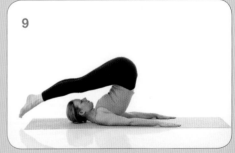

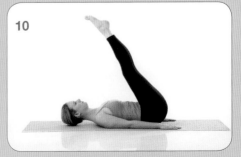

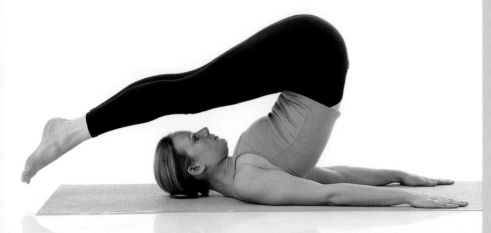

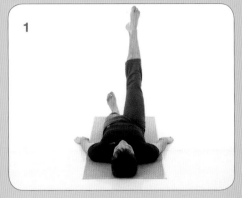

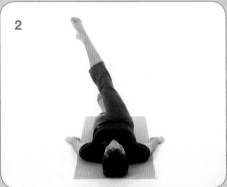

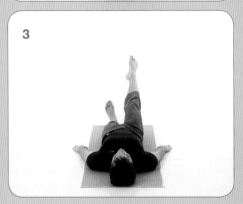

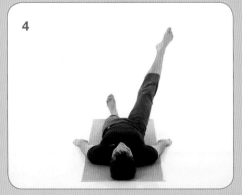

leg circles

Challenge the ability to move a lengthened leg freely from the hip, whilst ensuring that it moves independently from the pelvis and spine.

starting position

Align yourself correctly in the Relaxation Position. Fold your right leg in towards your body with stability and straighten it. Turn the leg out slightly from the hip and softly point your foot. Lengthen your left leg in parallel, straight along the mat, and flex your foot.

Maintain an appropriate level of connection to your centre throughout.

action

● Breathe in. Maintaining a still and stable pelvis, bring your right leg towards the mid-line of the body and up towards the left shoulder.
● Breathe out as you lower the leg down and circle it around and up, back to the Starting Position.

Repeat five times, and then reverse the direction:

● Breathe in as you reach the leg slightly out, as wide as the right shoulder.
● Breathe out as you lower the leg down and circle it around and up, back to the Starting Position.

Repeat five times.

To finish, lower the leg to the mat and repeat in both directions with the left leg.

WATCH POINTS

★ Keep your pelvis and spine stable and still throughout. Focus on the independent movement of the thigh bone in the hip socket.

★ Maintain a slight turn-out of the leg from the hip throughout the circle.

★ Fully lengthen both legs but avoid locking your knees.

rolling like a ball

Challenges the ability to maintain the integrity of a C-Curved spine.

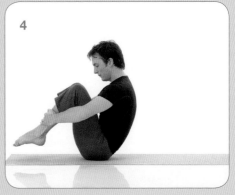

starting position

Sit in a C-Curve, with your pelvis rolled underneath you and your spine lengthening away from a strong and connected centre. Bend your knees, connect your heels and slightly open your knees. Circle your arms around the outside of your legs and take hold of your ankles. Lift your feet slightly off the mat, finding a balanced position.

Maintain an appropriate level of connection to your centre throughout.

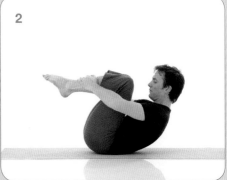

action

● Breathe in and, maintaining the curved shape of your spine, rock back onto your upper body. Carry the legs with you and balance briefly.

● Breathe out as you rock back with control to the Starting Position, once again ensuring that you maintain the relationship betwcen the legs and your spine. Repeat up to ten times.

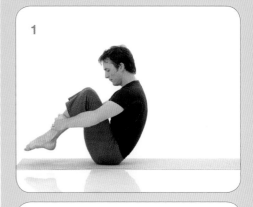

WATCH POINTS

★ Maintain the shape and length of the spine and the relationship between your spine and the legs as you roll.

★ Keep the waist long on both sides; avoid rotating to one side or side-bending. Connect your deep abdominals to support your spine.

★ Roll directly through your centre line, avoiding any deviations to either side.

★ Control the movement throughout: roll to the shoulders, not the head, and, as you roll forwards, do not let your feet touch the mat.

★ Breathe rhythmically to achieve the flowing movement required.

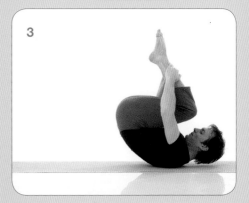

single leg stretch

Develops strength and stamina in the abdominal area while mobilising the hips and knees.

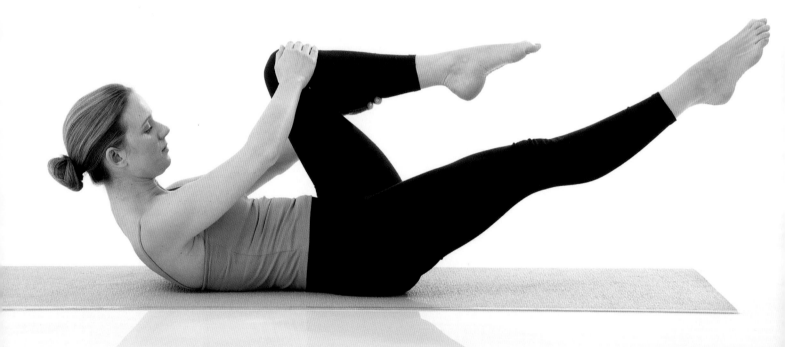

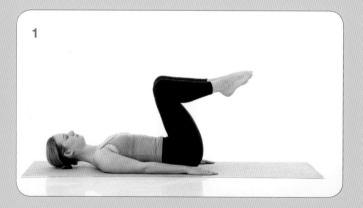

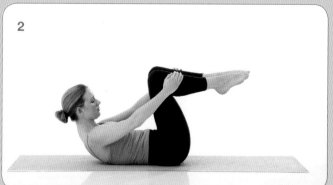

starting position

Align yourself correctly in the Relaxation Position. Double Knee Fold one leg at a time with stability and, keeping your heels connected and your feet softly pointed, open your knees slightly. (If performing the Advanced Matwork Sequence, connect your inner thighs and lift both legs off the mat at the same time.) Breathe in, preparing your body to move, and, as you breathe out, nod your head and sequentially wheel your neck and upper body off the mat into a Curl Up position. Lengthen your arms forwards and place your hands onto the outside of your shins. Maintain an appropriate level of connection to your centre throughout.

WATCH POINTS

★ Keep all your movements controlled, smooth and flowing.

★ Ensure that your pelvis remains grounded in neutral throughout. Move your legs independently from your pelvis and spine.

★ Maintain the curled-up position throughout. Use your arms to draw your legs towards you and not to pull your spine up further.

★ Maintain length in your neck, and keep your head still; focus down onto your abdominal area.

action

● Breathe into the back of your ribcage as you hold the Curl Up.

● Breathe out as you straighten your right leg forwards in line with the hip. Simultaneously place the right hand on the left knee and gently draw the left leg in towards your torso.

● Continue to breathe out as you switch legs, bending the right leg in and drawing it in towards your torso as you press the left leg away. Your left hand will now be positioned on the right knee and the right hand on the right shin.

● Breathe in as you repeat a further two leg stretches, first pressing your right leg away and then your left leg.
Repeat up to five times.

To finish, remain curled up as you bend both knees in towards your torso. Roll your upper spine and head back down to the mat and then, maintaining a stable pelvis, return your feet to the mat to end in the Relaxation Position.

(If performing the Advanced Matwork Sequence, remain curled up and bend both knees in to establish the Starting Position for the Double Leg Stretch.)

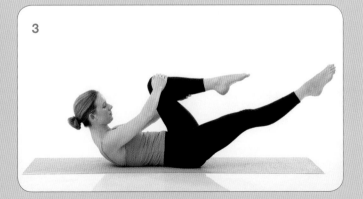

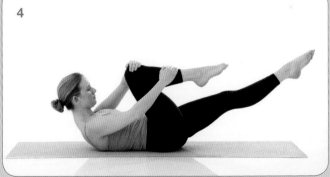

double leg stretch

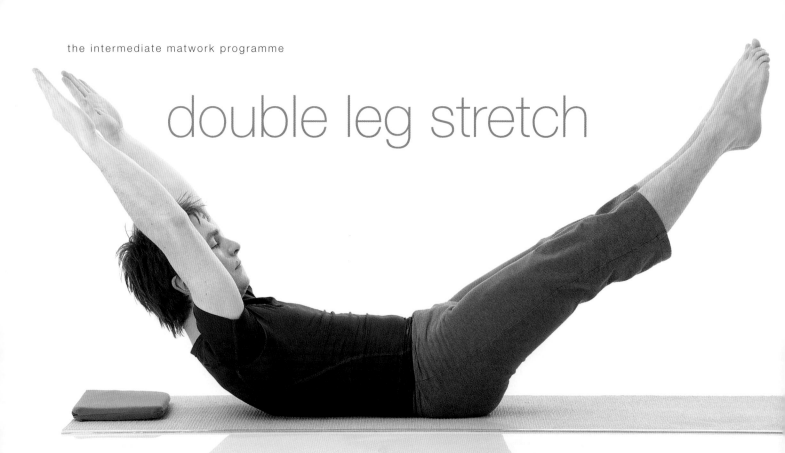

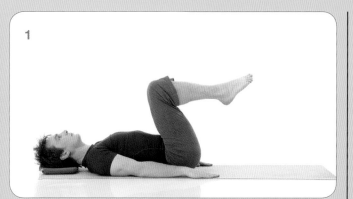

1

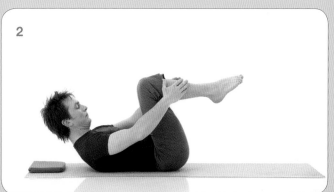

2

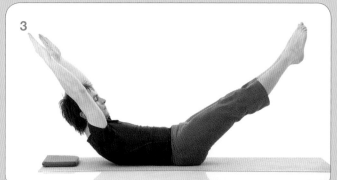

3

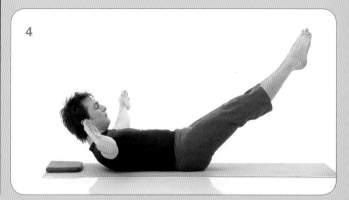

4

Develops strength and stamina in the abdominal area while mobilising the shoulders, hips and knees. Challenges coordination and control.

starting position

Align yourself correctly in the Relaxation Position. Double Knee Fold one leg at a time with stability and, keeping your heels connected and your feet softly pointed, open your knees slightly. (If performing the Advanced Matwork Sequence, connect your inner thighs and lift both legs off the mat at the same time.) Breathe in, preparing your body to move, and, as you breathe out, nod your head and sequentially wheel your neck and upper body off the mat into a Curl Up position. Lengthen your arms forwards and place your hands onto the outside of your shins. Maintain an appropriate level of connection to your centre throughout.

WATCH POINTS

★   Keep all of your movements controlled, smooth and flowing.

★   Ensure that your pelvis remains grounded in neutral throughout. Move your legs independently from your pelvis and spine.

action

● Breathe in, remaining curled up, and straighten both legs, pressing them away from your torso on a low diagonal. Connect your inner thighs in the Pilates Stance position. Simultaneously reach your straight arms overhead, shoulder-width apart.

● Breathe out as you bend the legs back in towards your torso, maintaining the connection of the heels as the knees open. Simultaneously circle the arms out to the side and around to return back to the shins and draw the legs back in to the Starting Position.

Repeat up to ten times.

To finish, roll your upper spine and head back down to the mat and then, maintaining a stable pelvis, return your feet to the mat to end in the Relaxation Position.

(If performing the Advanced Matwork Sequence, remain curled up to establish the Starting Position for Single Straight Leg Stretch.)

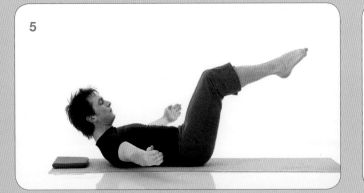

5

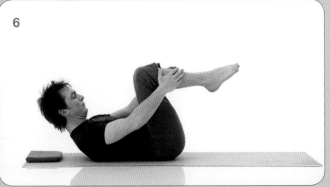

6

single straight leg stretch

Develops strength and stamina in the abdominal area while mobilising the hips with fully lengthened legs. Encourages precise and flowing movements.

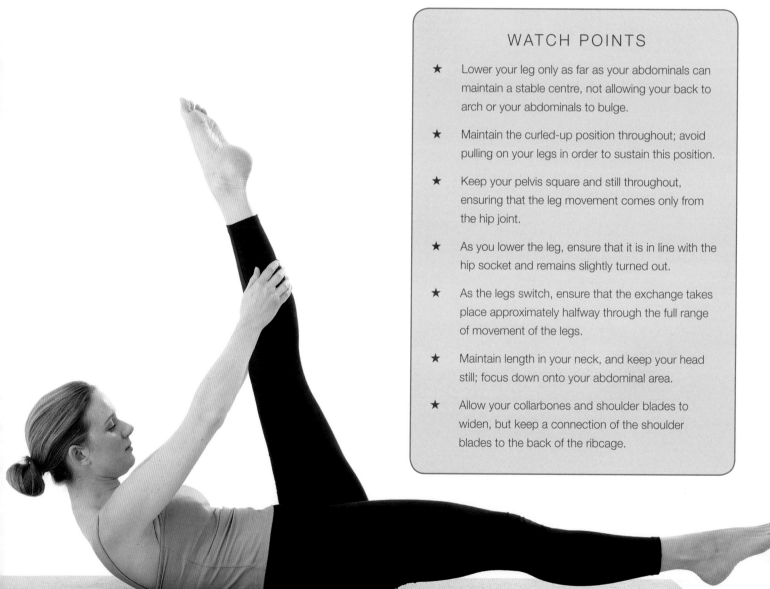

WATCH POINTS

★ Lower your leg only as far as your abdominals can maintain a stable centre, not allowing your back to arch or your abdominals to bulge.

★ Maintain the curled-up position throughout; avoid pulling on your legs in order to sustain this position.

★ Keep your pelvis square and still throughout, ensuring that the leg movement comes only from the hip joint.

★ As you lower the leg, ensure that it is in line with the hip socket and remains slightly turned out.

★ As the legs switch, ensure that the exchange takes place approximately halfway through the full range of movement of the legs.

★ Maintain length in your neck, and keep your head still; focus down onto your abdominal area.

★ Allow your collarbones and shoulder blades to widen, but keep a connection of the shoulder blades to the back of the ribcage.

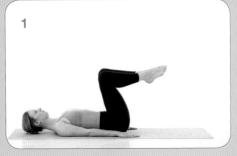

starting position

Align yourself correctly in the Relaxation Position. Double Knee Fold one leg at a time with stability and, keeping your heels connected and your feet softly pointed, open your knees slightly.

(If performing the Advanced Matwork Sequence, connect your inner thighs and lift both legs off the mat at the same time.)

Breathe in, preparing your body to move, and, as you breathe out, nod your head and sequentially wheel your neck and upper body off the mat into a Curl Up position. Simultaneously straighten your legs, connecting the inner thighs in Pilates Stance. Lengthening your arms, place both hands around your right calf or ankle. Your elbows are wide, ensuring that you remain open across the chest. Maintain an appropriate level of connection to your centre throughout.

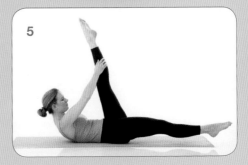

action

- Breathe into the back of your ribcage as you hold the curled-up position.
- Breathe out as you lower the left leg, stretching it out in line with the hip, about 8cm from the mat. Simultaneously pull the right leg towards you with a controlled double pulse, breathing 'out, out' as you do so. Maintain a stable and still pelvis and spine.
- Breathe in swiftly as you return the left leg back up; simultaneously begin to lower the right leg.
- Breathe out as you lower the right leg in line with the hip, just slightly off the mat. Simultaneously pull the left leg towards you with a controlled double pulse, once again breathing 'out, out' as you do so.

Repeat up to five times.

To finish, remain curled up as you bend both knees in towards your torso. Roll your upper spine and head back down to the mat and then, maintaining a stable pelvis, return your feet to the mat to finish in the Relaxation Position.

(If performing the Advanced Matwork Sequence, remain curled up with both legs straight and connected in Pilates Stance. Clasp your hands behind your head to establish the Starting Position for Double Straight Leg Raises).

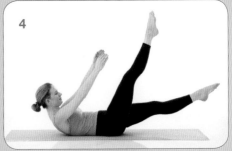

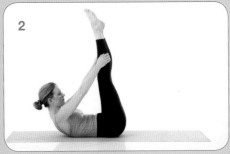

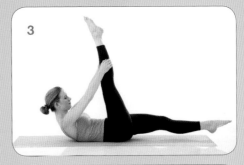

double straight leg raises

Develop strength and stamina in the abdominal area while mobilising the shoulders and hips with fully lengthened legs.

starting position

Align yourself correctly in the Relaxation Position. Double Knee Fold one leg at a time with stability and, keeping your heels connected and your feet softly pointed, open your knees slightly. Lightly clasp both hands behind your head, keeping the elbows open and positioned just in front of your ears within your peripheral vision.

(If performing the Advanced Matwork Sequence, connect your inner thighs and lift both legs off the mat at the same time.)

Breathe in, preparing your body to move, and, as you breathe out, nod your head and sequentially wheel your neck and upper body off the mat into a Curl Up position. Simultaneously straighten your legs, connecting the inner thighs in Pilates Stance.

Maintain an appropriate level of connection to your centre throughout.

action

- Breathe into the back of your ribcage as you hold the curled-up position and lower both legs away from your torso and down towards the mat as far as possible without arching or straining your back.
- Breathe in, maintaining a stable and still pelvis and a curled-up spine, as you return both legs towards the body with control. Repeat up to ten times.

To finish, remain curled up as you bend both knees in towards your torso. Roll your upper spine and head back down to the mat and then, maintaining a stable pelvis, return your feet to the mat to finish in the Relaxation Position.

(If performing the Advanced Matwork Sequence, remain curled up and bend both knees in to establish the Starting Position for Criss-cross.)

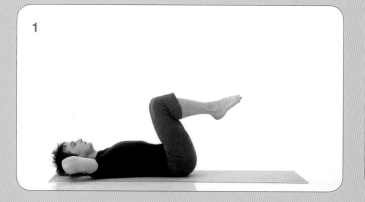

1

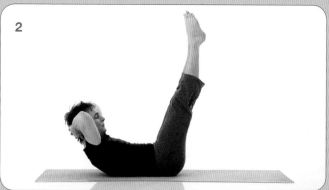

2

WATCH POINTS

★ Ensure that your pelvis remains grounded in neutral throughout; move your legs independently from your pelvis and spine.

★ Lower the legs only as far as your abdominals can maintain a stable centre, i.e. do not allow the back to arch or the abdominals to bulge.

★ Return the legs up only as far as your hamstrings will lengthen. Avoid allowing the pelvis to tilt towards you or the knees to bend.

★ Maintain length in your neck, and keep your head still; focus down onto your abdominal area.

★ Keep a connection of the shoulder blades to the back of the ribcage.

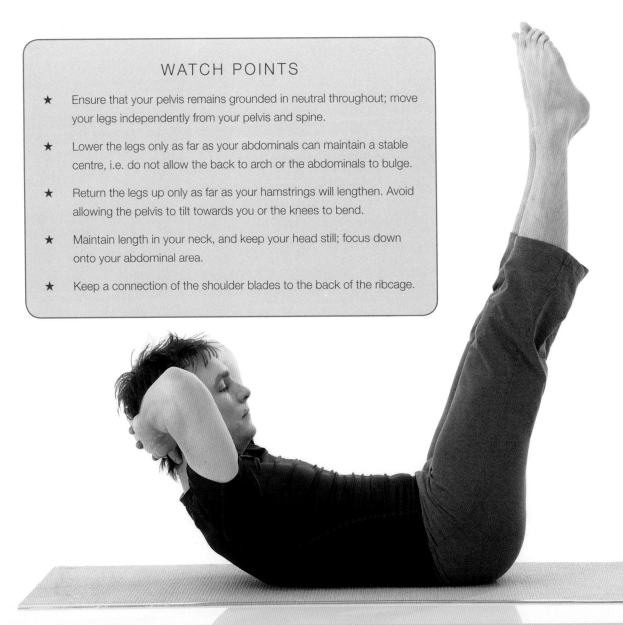

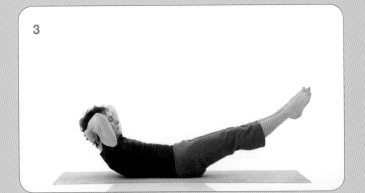

3

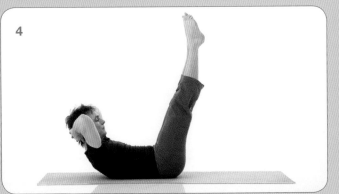

4

criss-cross

Develops strength and stamina in the abdominal area with a twisting motion of the torso, which demands precision, coordination and control.

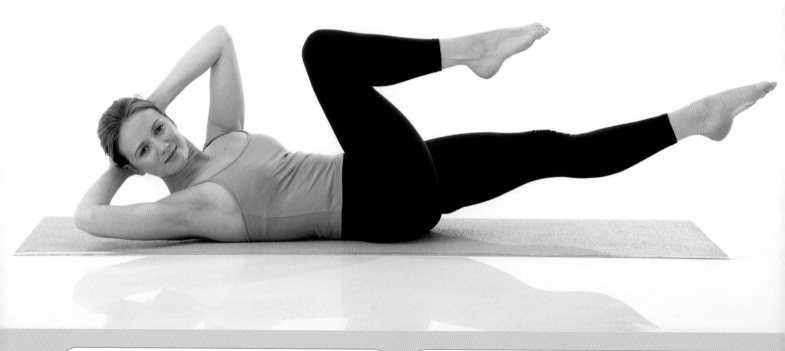

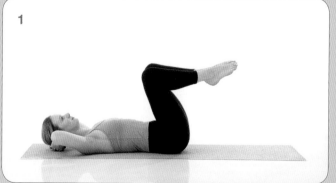

1

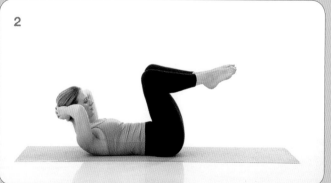

2

starting position

Align yourself correctly in the Relaxation Position. Double Knee Fold one leg at a time with stability and, keeping your heels connected and your feet softly pointed, open your knees slightly. Lightly clasp both hands behind your head, keeping the elbows open and positioned just in front of your ears within your peripheral vision.

(If performing the Advanced Matwork Sequence, connect your inner thighs and lift both legs off the mat at the same time.)

Breathe in, preparing your body to move, and, as your breathe out, nod your head and sequentially wheel your neck and upper body off the mat into a Curl Up position.

Maintain an appropriate level of connection to your centre throughout.

action

● Breathe into the back of your ribcage as you hold the curled-up position.

● Breathe out as you straighten and stretch your left leg away from you, simultaneously rotating your head and upper body to the right and drawing your right leg in further towards your torso.

● Breathe in as you draw your left leg back, whilst simultaneously stretching your right leg away and rotating your upper body to the left. Stay curled up.

Repeat up to five times.

To finish, remain curled up as you bend both knees in towards your torso. Remove your hands from behind your head and lengthen both arms forward, before rolling your upper spine and head back down to the mat. Maintaining a stable pelvis, return your feet to the mat to finish in the Relaxation Position.

(If performing the Advanced Matwork Sequence, connect your inner thighs and return both legs to the mat at the same time.

WATCH POINTS

★ As you rotate the spine from side to side, ensure that you stay curled up.

★ The rotation should come from the movement of the ribs on the spine and the spine itself. Try not to pull on your head.

★ Keep your pelvis square and still throughout, ensuring that the leg movement comes only from the hip joint.

★ Keep both sides of the waist equally long.

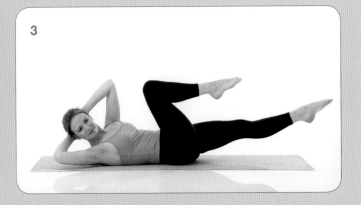

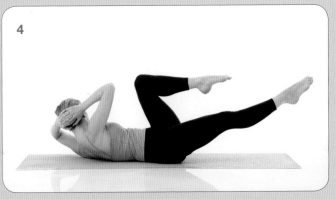

spine stretch forward

Aims actively to mobilise the entire spine, encouraging support from the deep abdominals. Reinforces awareness of lateral breathing.

starting position

Sit upright with your legs lengthened out in front of you; your pelvis and spine are in neutral, your legs are parallel, slightly wider than shoulder-width apart and your feet are flexed. Reach your arms out in front of you, slightly lower than shoulder height and shoulder-width apart. Your arms are lengthened, and your palms are facing down.

Maintain an appropriate level of connection to your centre throughout.

action

● Breathe in and lengthen your spine.
● Breathe out as you nod your head and begin to curl your spine forwards sequentially, wheeling vertebra by vertebra. Roll as far as is possible without disturbing the pelvis.
● Breathe in and, initiating from your centre, begin to roll your spine back up, re-stacking each vertebra until the pelvis, ribcage and head are once again vertically aligned.

Repeat up to five times, trying to deepen the curl each time.

WATCH POINTS

★ Your pelvis should remain still. Keep the weight even on both sitting bones and maintain their contact to the mat throughout.

★ Roll directly through your centre line.

★ Focus on connecting your deep abdominals to help support your spine as you roll forward and back up.

★ Use the breath pattern to emphasise your core connection and to increase your range of movement.

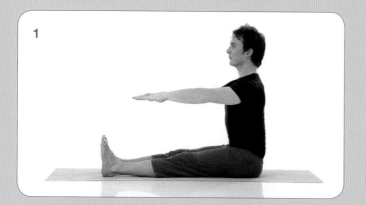

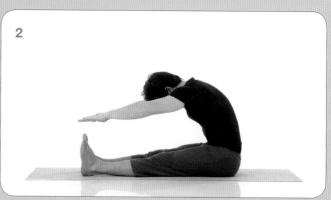

open leg rocker

Develops length in the spine while encouraging release along the back of the legs and challenging your balance and control.

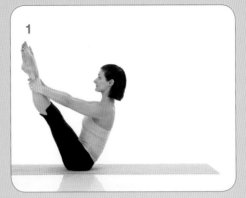

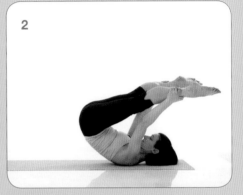

starting position

Sit in a C-Curve, with your pelvis rolled underneath you and your spine lengthening away from a strong and connected centre. Bend your knees, connect your heels and slightly open your knees. Circle your arms around the outside of your legs and take hold of your ankles. Lift your feet slightly off the mat and find a balanced position by lifting your chest, encouraging length through the upper back, neck and head; focus forward.

Breathe in and maintain the balanced position of your spine as you slowly extend both legs up into a 'V' position. Slightly turn out your legs from your hips, fully straightening your arms.

Maintain an appropriate level of connection to your centre throughout.

action

● Breathe out and, maintaining the relationship between the spine and the legs, rock back onto your upper body. Balance there briefly.

● Breathe in as you roll back smoothly to the upright 'V' position and again balance without altering the position of your spine.

Repeat up to five times.

To finish, bend your knees and lower your feet back to the mat with control.

WATCH POINTS

★ Maintain a constant position through the spine as you roll; the lower spine is slightly curved (but not collapsed) while the upper spine remains lifted and lengthened.

★ Avoid collapsing in any part of your body. Focus on connecting your deep abdominals to help support your spine.

★ Also maintain the relationship between the spine and the legs as you roll; the arms should remain straight.

★ Keep the arms straight throughout.

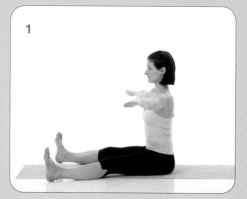

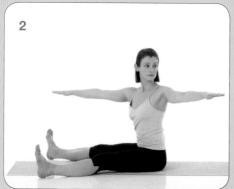

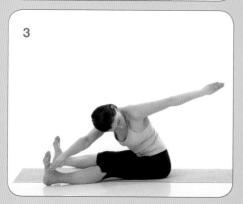

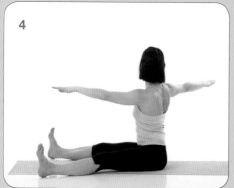

the saw

Mobilises the spine, in a similar way to the Spine Stretch Forward, but with added rotation, offering the opportunity to breathe fully.

starting position

Sit upright with your legs lengthened out in front of you; your pelvis and spine are in neutral. Your legs are parallel, slightly wider than shoulder-width apart, and your feet are flexed. Raise your arms out to the side of the body at shoulder height with your palms facing down.

Maintain an appropriate level of connection to your centre throughout.

action

● Breathe in as you fully rotate your head and body to the left.

● Breathe out as you curl the spine forwards over the left leg, leading with the head and maintaining the full rotation of your spine. Simultaneously reach the right arm across your left leg, palm facing down, and open the left shoulder joint as you reach the left arm behind and away in the opposite direction.

● Continue to breathe out fully as you pulse into your position three times, trying to deepen the position each time. Expel all of your breath on the very last pulse.

● Breathe in as you roll up through the spine and then rotate back through the Starting Position all the way through to the right.

● Breathe out as you curl the spine forwards over the right leg, leading with the head and maintaining the full rotation of the body and head. Simultaneously reach the left arm across the right leg, palm facing down, and open the right shoulder joint as you reach the right arm behind and away in the opposite direction.

● Continue to breathe out fully as you pulse into your position three times, trying to deepen the position each time. Expel all of your breath on the very last pulse. Repeat up to five times. Then return to the Starting Position in the centre.

WATCH POINTS

★ Keep your pelvis still and grounded throughout, ensuring that as you are rotating and reaching the opposite sitting bone does not lift off the mat.

★ Focus on connecting your deep abdominals to help support your spine as you rotate, roll and re-stack.

★ Keep reaching in opposite directions through both arms and continue to feel the openness across the front of the chest.

★ Fully lengthen both legs but avoid locking your knees.

★ Fully breathe; by the third pulse you should really feel that you are emptying your lungs. As you inhale fill the lungs up from the bottom to the top of the spine, coordinating this with the re-stacking of the spine.

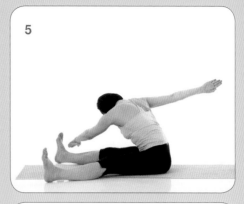

5

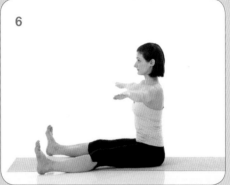

6

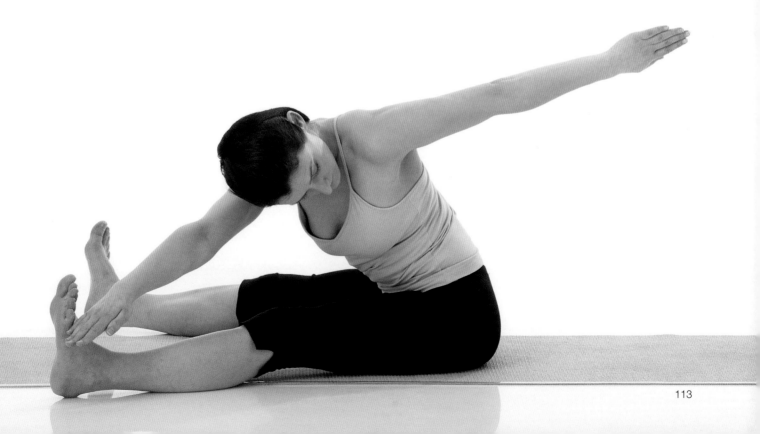

cobra

Promotes sequential mobilisation of the spine and hips, requiring strength in the back of the body balanced with mobility along the front of the body.

starting position

Lie on your front, correctly aligning your pelvis and spine in neutral, and rest your forehead on the mat. Your legs are straight, slightly wider than hip-width apart and turned out from the hips. Bend your elbows and position your hands slightly wider than and above your shoulders, with your palms facing down. Make sure that your shoulders are released and your collarbones are wide. Maintain an appropriate level of connection to your centre throughout.

WATCH POINTS

★ At the height of the Cobra, allow your hips to open and the front of your pelvis to lose contact with the mat. Keep your abdominals connected but lengthened.

★ Keep your legs straight and reaching away from the torso throughout.

action

● Breathe in as you begin to lengthen the front of the neck to roll and lift your head and continue to peel the front of the body smoothly off the mat: first the breastbone, then the ribcage and the abdominal area and finally the front of your pelvis. As the body wheels off the mat your arms will begin to straighten. Continue to lengthen the legs behind the body.

● Breathe out as you lower the spine down sequentially, maintaining length through the spine: first the front of your pelvis, then the abdominal area, the ribcage, breastbone and finally the head.

Repeat up to five times.

To finish, press up onto your hands and knees, and then fold back into the Rest Position (page 28) to allow your spine to release.

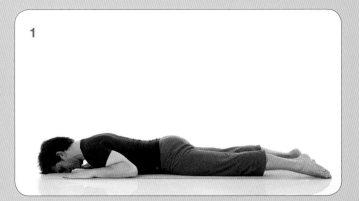

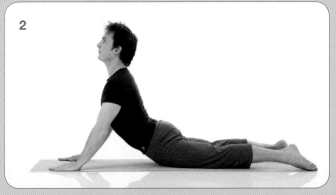

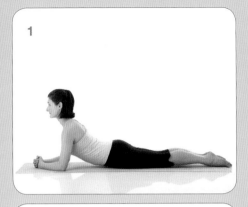

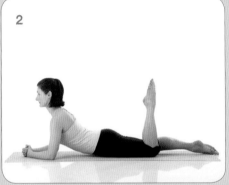

single leg kick

Develops strength in the buttocks, legs and spine while lengthening the front of the legs and hips; demands coordination and control.

starting position

Lie on your front; your legs are straight with the inner thighs connected together in parallel.

Bend your elbows, making a fist with one hand and clasping it with the other hand; your elbows are bent and slightly wider apart than your shoulders. Your spine is lengthened and extended, lifted off the mat. Open the front of your hips and also lift the front of your pelvis slightly off the mat. Open your chest and the front of your shoulders and focus forwards and slightly up.

Maintain an appropriate level of connection to your centre throughout.

action

● Breathe in, preparing your body to move, and lengthen your spine.

● Breathe out as you briskly kick the left heel towards the centre of your left buttock, toe softly pointed. Pulse twice, breathing 'out, out'.

● Straighten and stretch out your leg, returning it to the mat, and simultaneously kick your right foot towards your right buttock. Again pulse twice, breathing 'out, out'.

Repeat up to five times.

WATCH POINTS

★ Ensure that there is no compression or shortening of your lower spine; keep your abdominals connected but allow them to lengthen fully without collapse.

★ Maintain stability and stillness in your pelvis throughout, moving your legs independently from your pelvis and spine.

★ Your arms remain active throughout, anchoring down in order to keep the upper body lifted and the chest open.

★ Correct leg alignment is essential: hip, knee and ankle.

double leg kick

Strengthens the back muscles, using them to mobilise the head, neck and upper back, while also strengthening the backs of the legs.

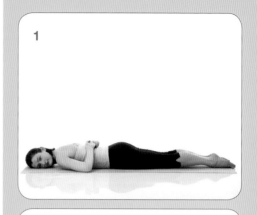

starting position

Lie on your front, correctly aligning your pelvis and spine in neutral; turn your head so that your right cheek is touching the mat. Your legs are straight and the inner thighs connected in parallel. Place your hands behind your back and clasp the right fingers (palm facing up) with the left hand and place them as far up your mid-back as is comfortable. Release the elbows as close to the mat as possible. Maintain an appropriate level of connection to your centre throughout.

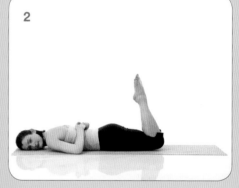

action

- Breathe in, preparing your body to move.
- Breathe out as you kick both legs towards your buttocks, keeping the legs together. Pulse three times: the accent is 'in, in, in'.
- Breathe in as you straighten the legs. Simultaneously, begin to lift and turn the head to the mat as your upper spine extends and your chest lifts away from the mat. Straighten the arms, reaching them down the body, turn your palms to face the back of your head and lift the arms slightly away from your buttocks.
- Breathe out and repeat the three kicks in. Simultaneously return your spine to the mat, turning your head to the right as the arms slide back up the body. (With each repetition, alternate the side towards which your head turns.)
Repeat up to five times.

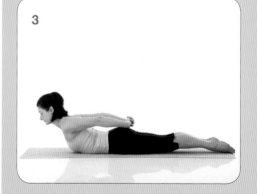

WATCH POINTS

★   As you lengthen the arms and legs away, ensure that you do not lock your knees or elbow joints.

★   As you return back down to the mat, do not collapse.

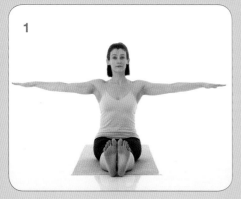

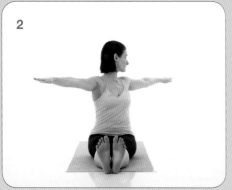

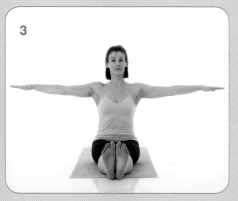

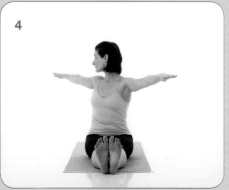

spine twist

Mobilises the head, neck and torso through a balanced rotational movement while challenging the stability of the pelvis and legs.

starting position

Sit upright with your legs lengthened out in front of you; your pelvis and spine are in neutral.

Your legs are parallel with the inner thighs connected and your feet are flexed.

Raise your arms out to the side of the body at shoulder height with your palms facing down.

Maintain an appropriate level of connection to your centre throughout.

action

● Breathe in, preparing your body to move, and lengthen your spine.

● Breathe out as you initiate a turn of the head and rotate your torso fully to the right. As you reach the end of the movement, pulse twice to increase your rotation, emptying the lungs fully.

● Breathe in as you lengthen and return to the Starting Position.

Repeat to the other side and then repeat the whole sequence up to five times.

WATCH POINTS

★   Your pelvis should remain still. Keep the weight even on both sitting bones and maintain their contact to the mat throughout.

★   Focus on connecting to your deep abdominals to help support your spine as you rotate and return.

★   The movement is pure rotation; continue to keep the spine lengthening vertically and avoid arching in your back or shortening in your waist.

★   Lengthen your arms and encourage width across the chest.

side kick series – front and back

Helps to mobilise and strengthen your hips while challenging your spinal stability.

WATCH POINTS

★ Avoid simply resting in the Starting Position but feel length and energy throughout your entire body.

★ Keep your chest open, and your focus directly ahead of you.

★ Ensure that your pelvis remains stable throughout. The action of the kick must come from your hip joint; your leg moves in isolation from the rest your body.

★ Be aware of your range of movement. The mobility in the hip joint and the flexibility of the surrounding muscles will dictate how far to carry the leg both forward and back. Do not allow movement to take place in the lower back.

★ The movement of the leg should be brisk but controlled.

★ Keep the underneath leg active; this will help you to balance.

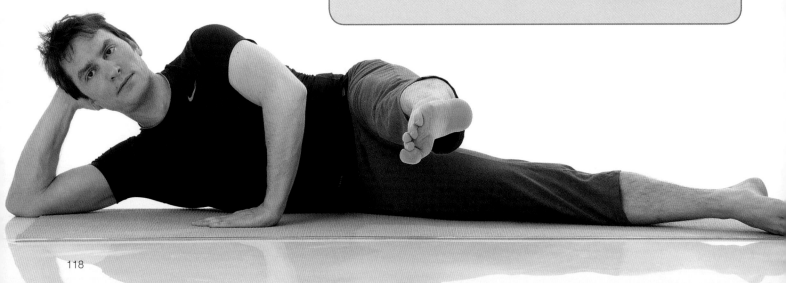

starting position

Lie on your right side, in a straight line, correctly stacking your shoulders, hips and ankles. Carry both legs forward, hinging from the hip joint, so that they are at an angle slightly in front of your body. Your pelvis and spine should remain in neutral. Prop your head up on your right arm, your elbow in line with your shoulder. Place your left hand behind your head with your elbow reaching towards the ceiling. Alternatively place your left hand on the mat in front of your ribcage and bend your elbow to help lightly support your position.

Lift your left leg so that it is level with the top of your pelvis. Keeping your pelvis still, reach the leg slightly behind you so that it is extended just behind the hip joint. Your leg remaining in parallel, softly point your foot.

Maintain an appropriate level of connection to your centre throughout.

action

● Breathe in as you sweep your left leg forward, hinging from the hip joint. The pelvis and spine remain stable. As you reach the end of the forward movement, draw your leg slightly back, flex the foot and then pulse it a little further forward.

● Breathe out as you point your foot and sweep the leg back again, to extend it just behind the hip joint.

Repeat up to ten times and then either continue with the Side Kick Series on the same side, or repeat on the other side.

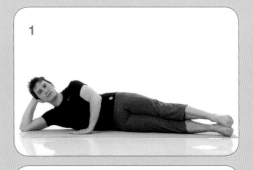

1

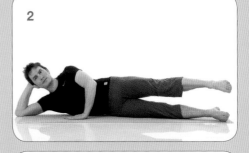

2

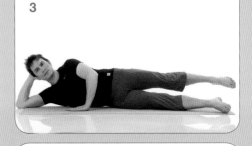

3

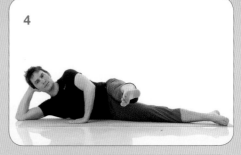

4

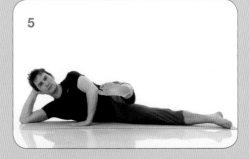

5

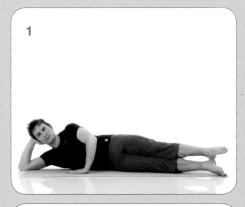

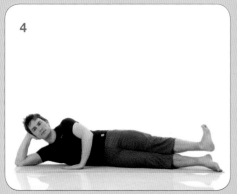

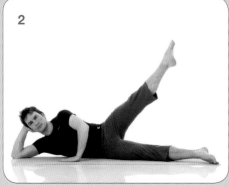

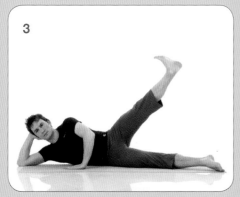

side kick series – up and down

starting position

Lie on your right side as before and, keeping your pelvis still, turn out your right leg from the hip and softly point your foot. Lengthen your legs and actively connect your inner thighs.

Maintain an appropriate level of connection to your centre throughout.

action

● Breathe in and, keeping your pelvis still, lengthen and lift your left leg directly up.

● Breathe out and flex your foot at the height of the kick, then slowly lower the leg back down to reconnect your inner thighs. Softly point your foot to prepare for the next kick.

Repeat up to ten times and then either continue with the Side Kick Series on the same side or repeat on the other side.

WATCH POINTS

★ Ensure that you constantly lengthen the leg away from you as kick it up and lower it down. Try to avoid 'hitching' your pelvis up towards your ribcage; keep the waist long.

★ Lift your leg directly up above the underneath leg and do not allow it to drift forward.

★ Avoid simply resting in the Starting Position but feel length and energy throughout your entire body.

★ Keep your chest open and your focus directly ahead of you.

★ Ensure that your pelvis remains stable throughout. The action of the kick must come from your hip joint; your leg moves in isolation from the rest your body.

side kick series – small circles

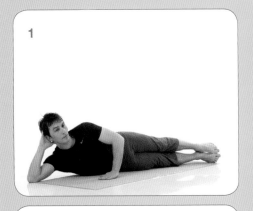

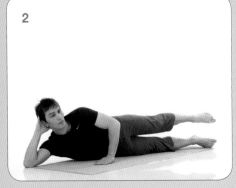

starting position

Lie on your right side as in the previous exercise.

Lift your left leg so that it is level with the top of your pelvis; your legs remain in parallel. Softly point your foot.

Maintain an appropriate level of connection to your centre throughout.

action

● Breathe in as you lengthen your left leg begin to circle it forward, down, back and up to the Starting Position.

● Breathe out. Perform another circle in the same direction.

● Repeat up to five times in the same direction (one breath for each circle) and then reverse direction.

Repeat up to ten times and then either continue with the Side Kick Series on the same side or repeat on the other side.

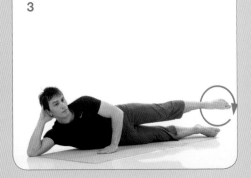

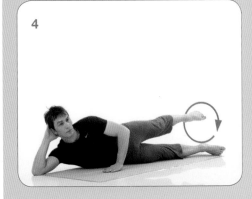

WATCH POINTS

★ The circle is small, about the size of a watermelon. Keep the circle even, i.e. as far as you carry the leg forward; you must carry it the same distance behind you.

★ Maintain the parallel position of your legs throughout the circle.

★ Avoid simply resting in the Starting Position but feel length and energy throughout your entire body.

★ Ensure that your pelvis remains stable throughout. The action must come from your hip joint, as your leg moves in isolation from the rest of your body.

★ Keep the underneath leg active; this will help your balance.

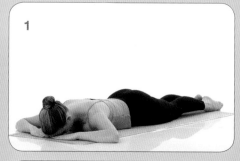

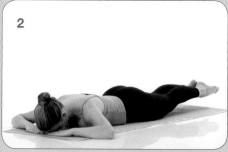

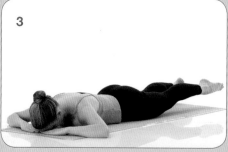

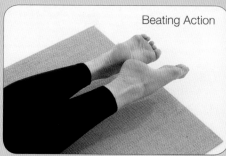

Beating Action

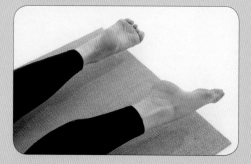

prone beats

Help to open up the front of the hips, while focusing on strengthening the back of the legs and the inner thighs.

starting position

Lie on your front, correctly aligning your pelvis and spine in neutral. Your legs are straight and the inner thighs connected in Pilates Stance. Create a diamond shape with the arms: place the fingertips together, palms down onto the mat, and open your elbows. Rest your forehead on the backs of the hands.

Breathe in, preparing your body to move, and, as you breathe out, lengthen and lift both legs slightly off the mat.

Maintain an appropriate level of connection to your centre throughout.

action

● Breathe in for a count of five as you open and close the inner thighs, beating them briskly together five times. The accent is 'in'.

● Breathe out for another count of five as you repeat the brisk beating action. Repeat up to three times.

WATCH POINTS

★ As you lift your legs off the mat, ensure that you do not disturb the stability and length of the pelvis and spine: they must remain in neutral.

★ Ensure that your pelvis remains stable and still throughout. The open and closing action of the legs must come from your hip.

★ The opening of the legs is small and the accent is 'in'.

★ Maintain the slight turn-out of your legs from the hips.

torpedo

Helps to mobilise and strengthen the hips and surrounding muscles while challenging spinal stability, balance and control.

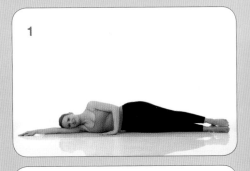

starting position

Lie on your right side in a straight line, correctly stacking your shoulders, hips and ankles. Lengthen your legs in line with your spine, connecting your inner thighs in parallel and softly pointing your feet. Your pelvis and spine remain in neutral. Lengthen your right arm underneath your head and in line with your spine. Place your left hand on the mat in front of your ribcage and bend your elbow to help lightly support your position.

Maintain an appropriate level of connection to your centre throughout.

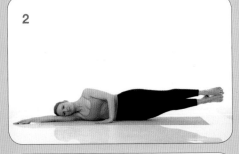

action

- Breathe in, preparing your body to move, and actively connect your inner thighs.
- Breathe out and, maintaining a stable and still pelvis and spine, raise both legs directly up off the mat. Keep your inner thighs connected.
- Breathe in, hold the position of the right leg and slightly raise your left leg even further.
- Breathe out and raise your right leg to join your left leg; connect the inner thighs.
- Breathe in and lower the connected legs with control back down to the mat. Repeat up to ten times.

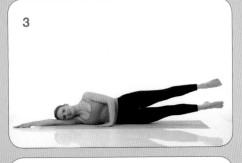

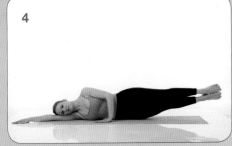

WATCH POINTS

★ Maintain length and energy throughout and keep your waist long.

★ Focus on balancing and avoid your spine rolling.

★ Avoid the legs drifting forwards or backwards and maintain their parallel alignment.

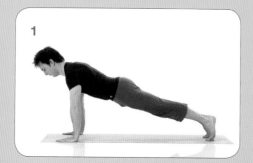

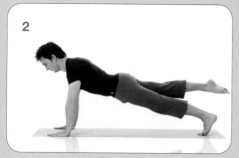

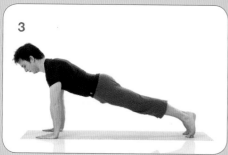

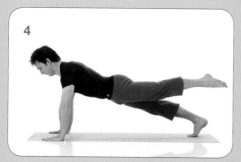

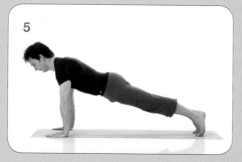

leg pull front

Challenges the stability of the spine and shoulder girdle.

starting position

Begin in a 'Plank' or 'Press Up' position: your arms are straight, hands directly underneath the shoulder joints and both legs are straight, with your inner thighs connected. Lift your heels and weight-bear through the balls of your feet. Your pelvis and spine are in neutral.

Maintain an appropriate level of connection to your centre throughout.

action

● Breathe in and, maintaining a stable and still pelvis, softly point your right foot, then lift your leg directly up. Simultaneously press your left heel towards the mat, stretching the back of the calf and shifting the weight of the body backwards slightly.

● Breathe out as you press forwards onto the ball of your left foot, returning the weight of the body forwards. Simultaneously lower your right leg and return the weight back to both legs.

Repeat three times and then repeat on the other side.

WATCH POINTS

★ It is essential to maintain a good abdominal connection to avoid your pelvis and spine dipping down towards the mat.

★ As you lift the leg up and behind the pelvis, ensure that you do so without disturbing the position of the pelvis or spine.

★ Focus on the opposition of your spine and legs throughout. For example, as you press your heel to the mat, continue to lengthen out through the crown of your head.

leg pull back

Requires a great deal of control and strength in the upper body to maintain a stable torso while mobilising and strengthening the hips.

starting position

Sit upright with your legs lengthened out in front of your body, inner thighs connected and feet softly pointed. Straighten your arms and circle them behind your body, to place the palms on the mat, fingers facing forwards.

Breathe in, preparing your body to move, and, as you breathe out, maintain a strong and stable centre, support the weight of the body with your arms and raise your pelvis off the mat to create a long diagonal line between the torso and the legs. Your hands and your heels remain on the floor, bearing weight. Lengthen your pelvis and spine into a neutral position but direct your focus forwards.

action

● Breathe in and lift the left leg directly upwards, keeping it straight. Keep your pelvis and spine stable and still.

● Breathe out and, at the height of the kick, flex your foot and lower your leg with control. Touch your foot to the mat but do not replace any weight. Softly point your foot.

Repeat the lift-and-lower of the right leg three times and then repeat three times on the left leg.

To finish, maintaining a strong centre, lower your pelvis back down to the mat.

WATCH POINTS

★ Keep your pelvis square and stable and the spine lengthened. Move your legs independently from your pelvis and spine.

★ Lift the weight of your body away from your arms and keep the front of your shoulders and your chest open.

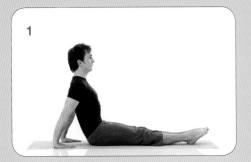

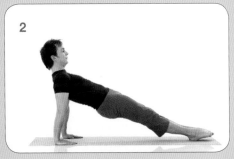

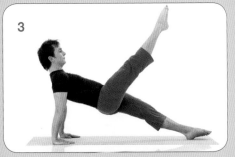

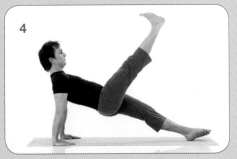

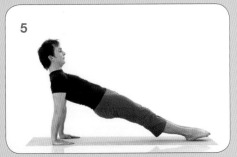

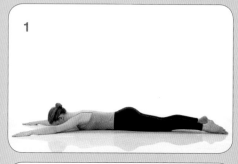

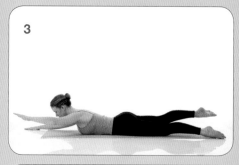

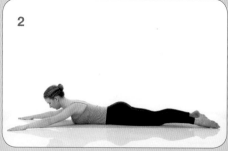

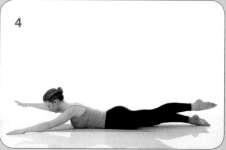

star

Develops an awareness of the independent movement of the arms and legs while the upper spine is stable and extended.

starting position

Lie on your front, correctly aligning your pelvis and spine in neutral, and rest your forehead on the mat. Your legs are straight, slightly wider than hip-width apart and turned out from the hips. Reach both arms above your head, slightly wider than shoulder-width and resting on the mat, your palms facing down.

Breathe in, preparing your body to move, and, as you breathe out, lift your head and chest slightly off the mat to extend your upper spine.

Maintain an appropriate level of connection to your centre throughout.

action

● Breathe in and lengthen your lifted spine. Keep your ribs in contact with the mat.
● Breathe out and, maintaining the position and stability of the spine, raise one arm and the opposite leg slightly off the mat.
● Breathe in as you lower your arm and leg back down to the mat, again maintaining the lift and length of the upper body.
Repeat up to ten times, alternating arms and legs.

WATCH POINTS

★ Ensure that there is no compression or shortening of your lower spine; keep your abdominals connected but allow them to lengthen fully without collapse.

★ Raise your arm and leg only as high as you can maintain a stable and still pelvis and spine.

★ Keep your chest lifted away from the mat and the chest open.

seal

Challenges your ability to maintain the integrity of a C-Curved spine. Massages the spine while maintaining a strong centre.

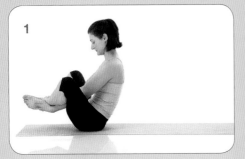

starting position

Sit in a C-Curve, with your pelvis rolled underneath you and your spine lengthening away from a strong and connected centre. Bend your knees and turn your legs out from the hips so that you can press the soles of your feet together. Weave your arms through the insides of your legs and wrap your hands around the outsides of the ankles. Maintaining this shape, lift your feet slightly off the mat, finding a balanced position.

Maintain an appropriate level of connection to your centre throughout.

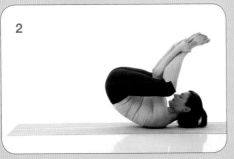

action

● Breathe in and, maintaining the curved shape of your spine, rock back onto your upper body; carry the legs with you. Balance briefly and clap the soles of your feet together three times, opening and closing from the hips.

● Breathe out as you rock back smoothly to the Starting Position once again, ensuring that you maintain the relationship between the legs and your spine. Balancing with your feet lifted slightly off the mat, again clap the soles of your feet together three times. Repeat the whole sequence up to five times.

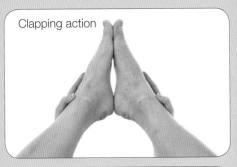

Clapping action

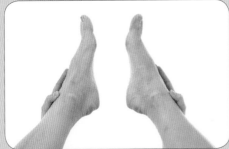

WATCH POINTS

★ Maintain the shape of the spine and the relationship between your spine and the legs as you roll. Keep the waist long on both sides.

★ Focus on the length of the spine whilst still maintaining the C-Curve; connect your deep abdominals to support your spine.

★ Open and close from your hips as you clap the feet.

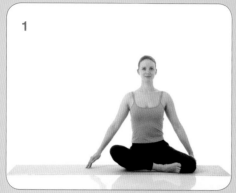

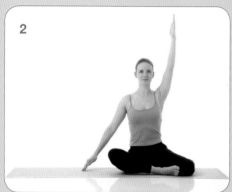

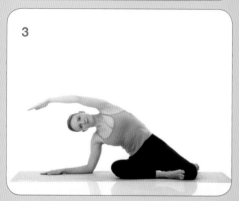

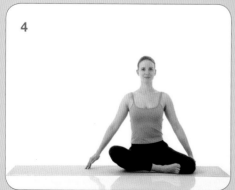

mermaid

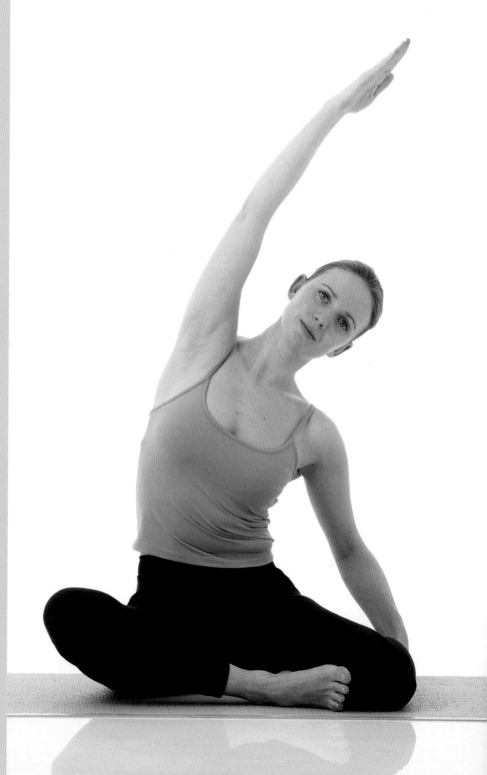

Promotes release along the sides of the body by mobilising the spine in side flexion; also helps to encourage lateral breathing.

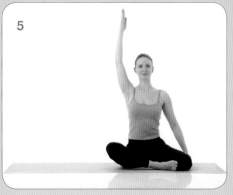

starting position

Kneel on the mat, sitting back onto your heels. Then move your pelvis off the heels to the right and onto the mat. If necessary, you may need to open your knees slightly, in order to find a comfortable position. Place your left hand onto your left ankle; your right hand is placed on the mat beside your pelvis. Encourage your pelvis to be as level as possible, although the left sitting bone will be slightly lifted. Lengthen and lift your spine from a strong centre.
Maintain an appropriate level of connection to your centre throughout.

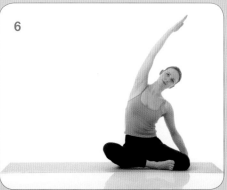

action

- Breathe in as you raise your left arm out to the side and overhead.
- Breathe out as you reach up and over, side-bending your spine to the right. Maintain the relationship between the left arm and your head. Your right arm will reactively slide further along the mat and then bend, so that your forearm can support your position.
- Breathe in. Maintain the length and position of your spine and focus on breathing laterally.
- Breathe out as you straighten the right arm and return the spine back to the vertical position. Lower your left arm and return your hand to your ankle.
- Breathe in as you raise the right arm overhead.
- Breathe out as you reach up and over, side-bending your spine, this time to the left. Again reach your right arm with your spine; use your left arm to encourage your spine over into the side-bend but keep lengthening up as you go over.
- Breathe in to maintain the position and focus on breathing laterally.
- Breathe out as you return to the upright position and lower the arms to the Starting Position.
Repeat up to five times.

WATCH POINTS

★ As you side-bend, initiate the movement with your head, followed sequentially with your ribcage. As you return, initiate the movement from your centre.

★ The side bend should be a lengthened position; avoid any compression and feel support from the abdominals.

★ Ensure that you have moved in one plane only and not curved forward or arched back.

★ Keep your head and neck in line with the rest of your spine.

workouts

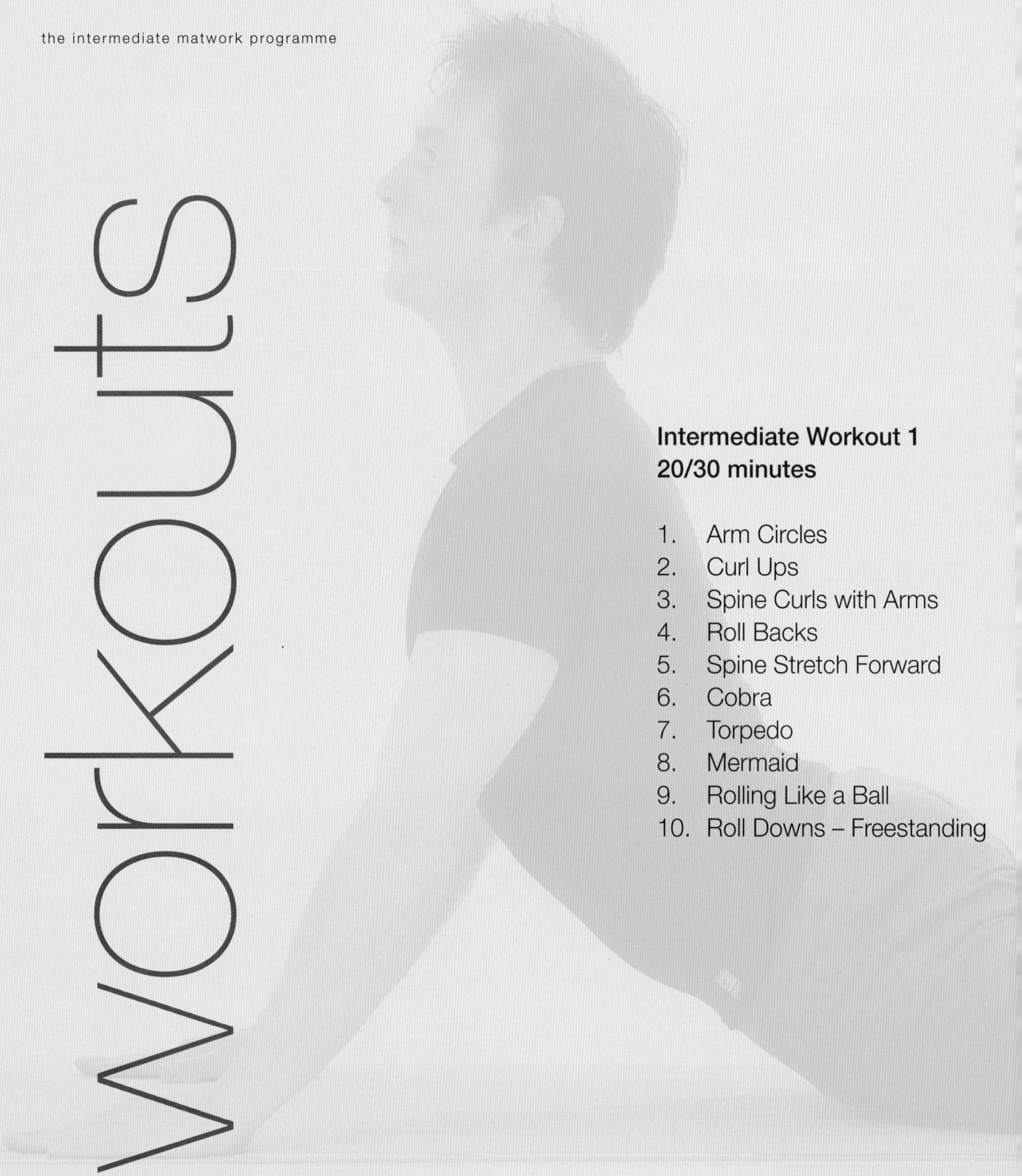

**Intermediate Workout 1
20/30 minutes**

1. Arm Circles
2. Curl Ups
3. Spine Curls with Arms
4. Roll Backs
5. Spine Stretch Forward
6. Cobra
7. Torpedo
8. Mermaid
9. Rolling Like a Ball
10. Roll Downs – Freestanding

Intermediate Workout 2
40/50 minutes

1. Spine Stretch Forward
2. Roll Backs
3. The Hundred
4. Roll Up
5. Roll Over
6. Single Leg Stretch
7. Double Leg Stretch
8. Criss-cross
9. Spine Stretch Forward
10. The Saw
11. Cobra
12. Single Leg Kick
13. Side Kick Series – Front and Back
14. Side Kick Series – Up and Down
15. Star
16. The Cat
17. Rest Position
18. Floating Arms
19. Tennis Ball Rising

Intermediate Workout 3
60/70 minutes

1. Ribcage Closure
2. Curl Ups
3. The Hundred
4. Roll Up
5. Roll Over
6. Leg Circles
7. Rolling Like a Ball
8. Single Leg Stretch
9. Double Leg Stretch
10. Single Straight Leg Stretch
11. Criss Cross
12. Spine Stretch Forward
13. Open Leg Rocker
14. The Saw
15. Cobra
16. Double Leg Kick
17. Spine Twist
18. Side Kick Series – Front and Back
19. Side Kick Series – Up and Down
20. Side Kick Series – Small Circles
21. Prone Beats
22. Leg Pull Front
23. Mermaid
24. Seal
25. Roll Downs – Freestanding

Chapter Four:
The Advanced
Matwork Programme

Here we have included the final and most challenging of the Pilates matwork exercises.

Study the exercises carefully and attempt them only when you feel strong and confident at performing the Intermediate exercises outlined in Chapter Three. It may take years of practice and understanding to master these exercises, so approach it as a progressive journey and enjoy the process.

Once you feel ready, you should try the Advanced Matwork Sequence, which is explained on page 166.

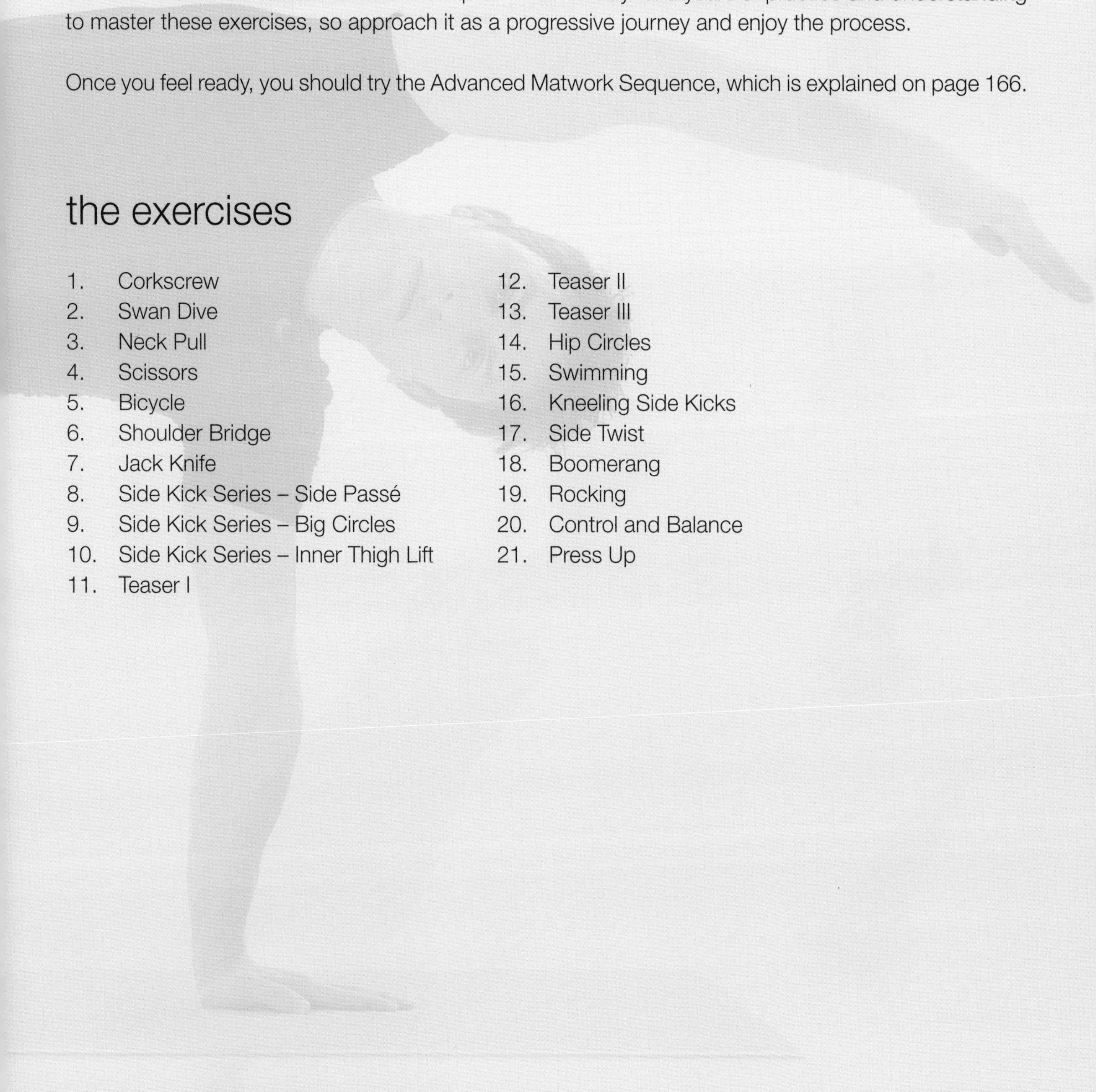

the exercises

1. Corkscrew
2. Swan Dive
3. Neck Pull
4. Scissors
5. Bicycle
6. Shoulder Bridge
7. Jack Knife
8. Side Kick Series – Side Passé
9. Side Kick Series – Big Circles
10. Side Kick Series – Inner Thigh Lift
11. Teaser I

12. Teaser II
13. Teaser III
14. Hip Circles
15. Swimming
16. Kneeling Side Kicks
17. Side Twist
18. Boomerang
19. Rocking
20. Control and Balance
21. Press Up

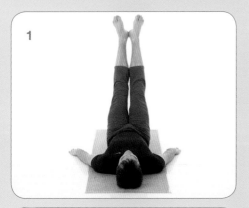

1

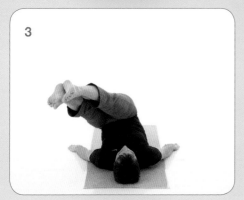

2

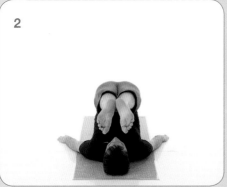

3

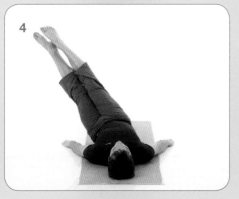

4

corkscrew

Promotes sequential mobilisation of the hips and spine, requiring much balance and strength throughout the whole body.

WATCH POINTS

★ Initiate the movement from a strong centre. Use the breath and avoid momentum.

★ Avoid rolling too far over.

★ Keep the pelvis lifting away from your ribcage to maintain length.

★ Avoid hitching or twisting as the spine rolls.

★ Keep your neck long, your chest open and the arms long on the mat.

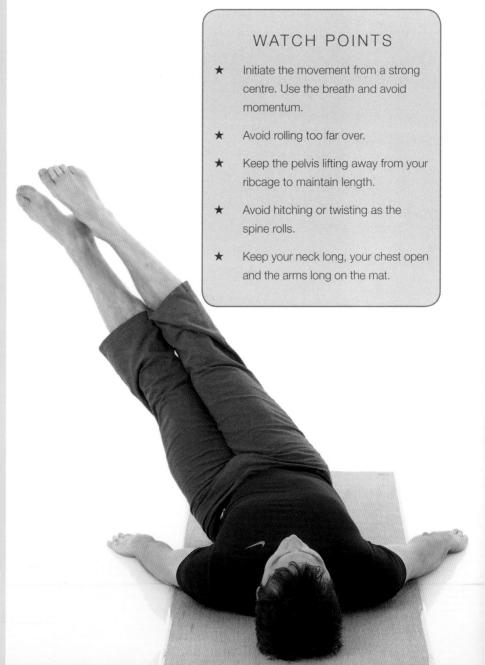

starting position

Advice: Before you attempt this exercise ensure that you have mastered the following exercises: Hip Rolls, Roll Over.

Align yourself correctly in the Relaxation Position. Connect your inner thighs together and Double Knee Fold both legs in towards you. Straighten both legs directly above your pelvis, turn them out into Pilates Stance and then lower them to a point where you can still maintain a neutral pelvis and spine; do not allow your lower back to arch.

Maintain an appropriate level of connection to your centre throughout.

The movement is continuous, flowing and dynamic without momentum. The breathing pattern is essential to achieving this.

action

- Breathe in as you lengthen the legs and begin to draw them in towards your body; keep your pelvis down for as long as possible.
- Breathe out as you allow your pelvis and spine to roll sequentially off the mat, drawing the legs up and over your torso until they are parallel with the mat. Make sure that you do not roll too far – there should not be any pressure on the neck and head or tension in the shoulders.
- Breathe in and reach the legs to the left allowing the pelvis and the spine to roll slightly. Keeping the legs directed to the left, begin to roll down the left side of your spine.
- Breathe out as you complete the roll, imprinting your lower spine and the back of the pelvis into the mat. Lower your legs and circle them to arrive at the centre line of the body slightly lower than vertical – the pelvis and spine are once again in neutral.
- Continue to breathe out, and circle your legs to the right. Draw the legs in towards your body and begin to roll up the right side of your spine.
- Once the spine has rolled to the base of the shoulder blades, circle the legs to the centre line of the body.

Repeat three times, reversing the direction of the circle each time.

To finish, keep the legs centred and roll your spine one vertebra at a time down onto the mat. Bend both knees and keep the inner thighs connected and the pelvis stable. Lower the legs back down to the mat.

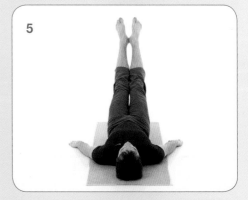

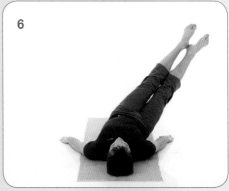

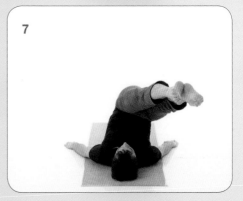

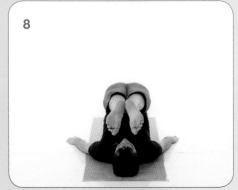

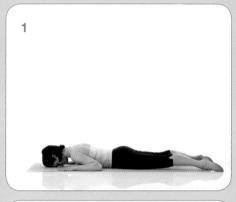

1

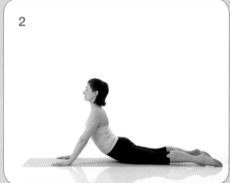

2

swan dive

Strengthens the back of the spine and legs while promoting openness in the front of the spine and legs.

starting position

Lie on your front, correctly aligning your pelvis and spine in neutral, and rest your forehead on the mat. Your legs are straight, slightly wider than hip-width apart and turned out from the hips. Bend your elbows and position your hands slightly wider than and in front of your shoulders, your palms facing down. Make sure that your shoulders are released and your collarbones are wide.

Breathe in as you begin to lengthen the front of the neck to roll and lift your head, continuing to peel the front of the body off the mat smoothly: first the breastbone, then the ribcage and the abdominal area and finally the front of your pelvis. As the body wheels off the mat your arms will begin to straighten. Continue to lengthen the legs behind the body.

Perform three repetitions of Cobra (page 114) before you begin Swan Dive. Maintain an appropriate level of connection to your centre throughout.

The goal of this exercise is to find the lengthened and arched shape of the arms, spine and legs and to maintain this position as you rock forwards and back.

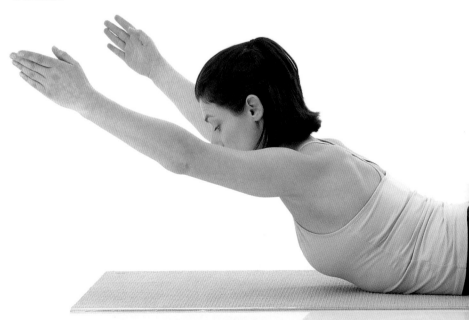

action

● Maintain the lengthened and arched shape of the spine as you reach your arms forwards, straight and in line with your ears, and rock forwards onto your ribcage. At the same time lift both legs off the mat, lengthening and lifting the legs straight behind you.

● Breathe in and rock back, lifting the chest high and keeping the arms lengthening up. Press the legs down and lengthen them behind you.
Repeat up to five times.

To finish, press up onto your hands and knees and then fold back into the Rest Position (page 28) to allow your spine to release.

WATCH POINTS

★ Ensure that there is no compression or shortening of your lower spine. Keep your abdominals connected but allow them to lengthen fully without collapse.

★ Emphasise the lift of the legs during the rock forwards and the pressing down of the legs during the rock up.

★ Always keep the legs straight and reaching away in opposition to the spine.

★ Remain long in the neck and avoid throwing the head back as you rock up or dropping it forwards as you rock down. The head moves with the spine.

★ Keep the arms lengthening by the side of your head but try to avoid over-elevating the shoulders.

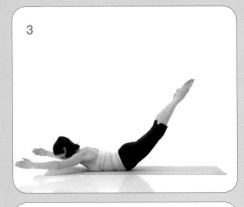

3

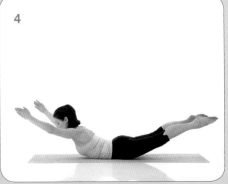

4

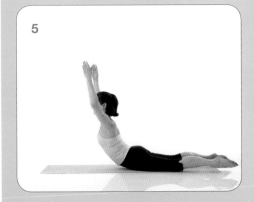

5

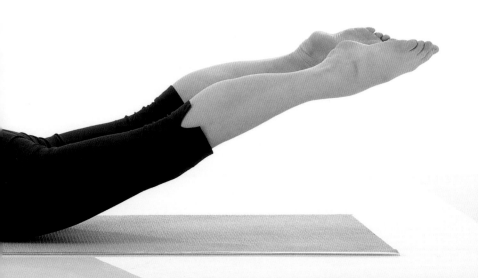

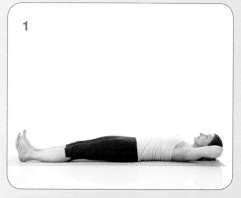

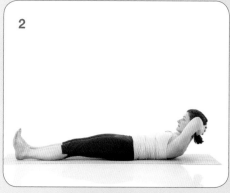

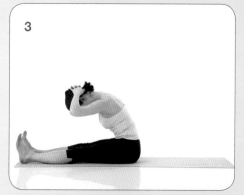

neck pull

Promotes sequential mobilisation of the spine and hips and challenges the balance of strength and mobility throughout the body.

starting position

Advice: Ensure that you have mastered Roll Up before attempting Neck Pull.
Lie on your back with both legs straight, hip-width apart and parallel, and your feet flexed. Your pelvis and spine are in neutral. Lightly clasp both hands behind your head, keeping the elbows open and fairly wide.
Maintain an appropriate level of connection to your centre throughout.
This exercise requires you to focus on your breath and keep the whole movement even-paced and flowing.

action

● Breathe in as you lengthen the back of your neck and nod your head forwards and sequentially curl up the upper body.
● Breathe out as you continue to wheel the spine one vertebra at a time off the mat. Curl smoothly and with control. Keeping the elbows wide, lengthen the curled spine over the legs.
● Breathe in as you re-stack the spine rolling up from your centre to the crown of your head. As you draw your body up, lengthen the legs away from your spine, pressing the heels forwards. Also encourage a gentle stretch through the back of the neck.
● Breathe out as you emphasise the deep connection of the abdominals and curl the pelvis underneath you. Keeping the elbows wide, lengthen your head and chest away as the spine rolls one vertebra at a time onto the mat. Finally roll the shoulders and head back down onto the mat.
Repeat up to five times.

WATCH POINTS

★ Ensure that you roll smoothly through each segment of your spine, articulating on the way up and on the roll down.

★ Beware not to curl forwards excessively from the head and neck – remember you are still looking for a balanced C-Curve shape in the spine.

★ Roll directly through your centre line, avoiding any deviations to either side.

★ Keep your elbows wide throughout the exercise. Do not pull them in to help you roll up.

★ Keep a relationship between the shoulders and the back of your ribcage. Neither force them to depress, nor allow them to over-elevate, especially while rolling forwards.

★ Your spine will move with more ease if you keep the legs grounded down and lengthening away.

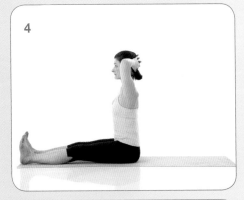

4

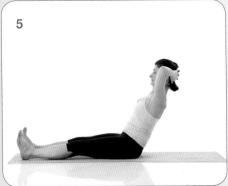

5

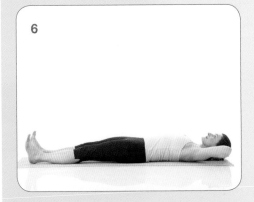

6

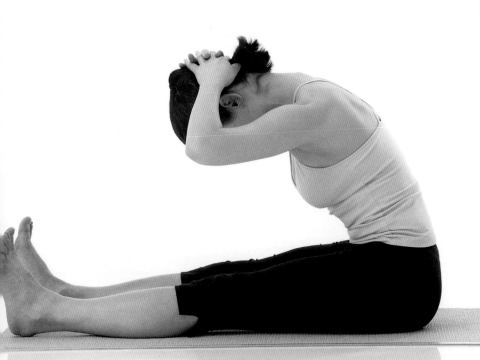

scissors

Promotes pelvic and spinal stability while mobilising the hips through a full range of movement, requiring a great deal of awareness, control and balance.

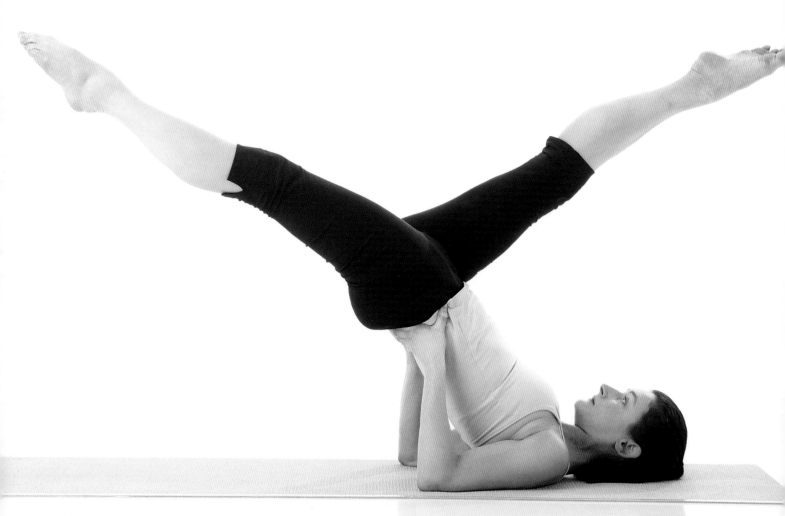

starting position

Align yourself correctly in the Relaxation Position. Connect your inner thighs together and Double Knee Fold both legs in towards you. Straighten both legs directly above your pelvis and softly point your feet.

Breathe in, preparing your body to move and, as you breathe out, begin to draw the legs in towards your body, curl the pelvis and then peel the spine one vertebra at a time off the mat.

Breathe in, place your hands on the back of your pelvis for support and press your pelvis and legs directly up to the ceiling. Press your upper arms gently down into the mat and keep your chest wide and open.

Maintain an appropriate level of connection to your centre throughout.

Focus on maintaining a still pelvis and strong centre throughout. Keep the legs lengthening up and away from the spine as they scissor.

action

● Breathe out as you split the legs, reaching one leg forward toward the mat while the other leg reaches over your head.

● Continuing to breathe out, scissor the legs, reaching the other leg forwards and drawing the opposite leg towards you. Your legs should pass one another directly above the pelvis.

● Breathe in and continue to scissor the legs forwards and backwards.

Repeat three times.

To finish, either connect the legs together and then continue with Bicycle (page 142) or lower the legs overhead and slowly and sequentially begin to roll your spine back down to the mat and reach your legs above your pelvis. Bend both knees and, keeping the inner thighs connected, lower the legs back down to the mat.

WATCH POINTS

★ Focus on the opposition between your legs and the spine. Avoid the weight of your body resting either on your hands or your neck. Your hands should be supporting the pelvis but the connection of your abdominals, inner thighs and buttocks will help to maintain the stability of your position.

★ As your reach the legs away from one another, focus on stretching the back of the leg that is overhead and the hip and the front of the leg that is reaching forwards.

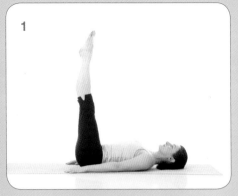

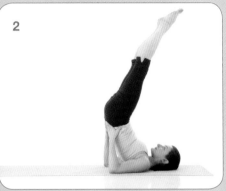

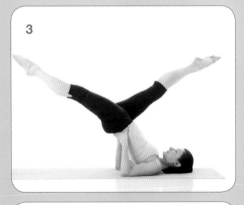

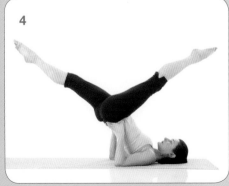

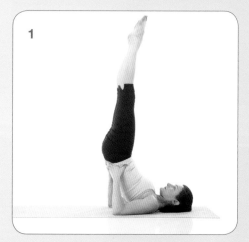

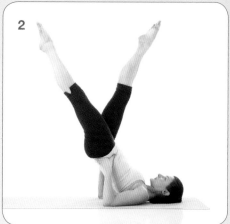

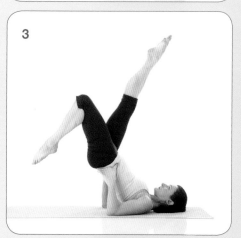

bicycle

Promotes pelvic and spinal stability while mobilising the hips and knees with a great deal of awareness, control and balance.

starting position

Remain in the position for Scissors (page 140) and draw the legs together, reaching them above the pelvis.

OR

Align yourself correctly in the Relaxation Position. Connect your inner thighs together and Double Knee Fold both legs in towards you. Straighten both legs directly above your pelvis and softly point your feet.

Breathe in, preparing your body to move, and, as you breathe out, begin to draw the legs in towards your body, curl the pelvis and then peel the spine one vertebra at a time off the mat. Breathe in, place your hands on the back of your pelvis for support and press your pelvis and legs directly up to the ceiling. Press your upper arms gently down into the mat and keep your chest wide and open.

Maintain an appropriate level of connection to your centre throughout.

This exercise challenges coordination and correct timing is essential. Try to straighten one leg at the same time as you are bending the other leg.

WATCH POINTS

★ Focus on the opposition between your legs and the spine. Avoid the weight of your body resting either on your hands or your neck. Your hands should be supporting the pelvis, but the connection of your abdominals, inner thighs and buttocks will help to maintain the stability of your position.

★ Reach the straight leg up to the ceiling – this requires a lot of balance and core control. Try not to let this leg drop down towards your face.

★ Ensure correct alignment of the legs, especially as they are bending. Both the ankle and knee should remain in line with your hip.

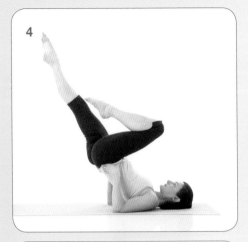

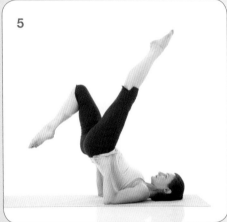

action

- Breathe out, engage your deep core muscles and reach the right leg to the ceiling as you reach the left leg forwards towards the mat.
- Bend the left knee, drawing the heel towards your buttock.
- Keeping the left leg bent, draw the leg back until your knee is above your hip. At the same time keep the right leg straight and reach it forward.
- Breathe in as you bend the right knee and at the same time straighten the right leg, directing it upwards.
- Draw the bent right leg in towards your body and reach the straight left leg forwards.
- Breathe out as you straighten the leg above your pelvis and bend the left knee, heel towards the buttock.

Repeat three sets and then reverse the direction of the Bicycle.

To finish, connect the legs together, lower them overhead and then slowly and sequentially begin to roll your spine back down to the mat and reach your legs above your pelvis. Bend both knees and, keeping the inner thighs connected, lower the legs back down to the mat.

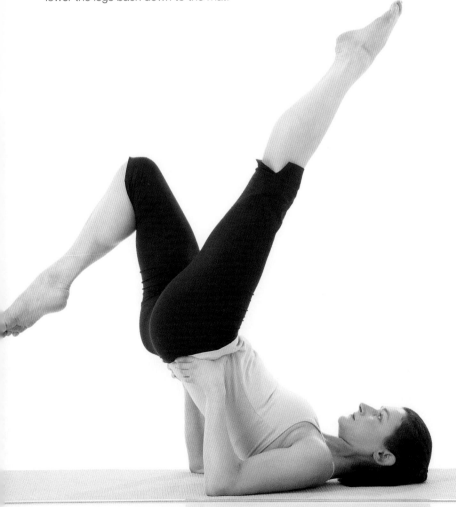

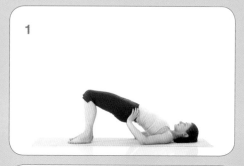

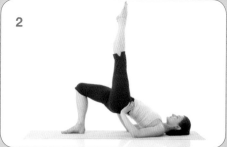

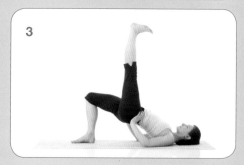

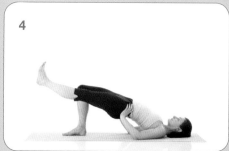

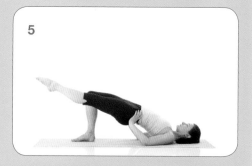

shoulder bridge

Develops spinal mobility as well as pelvic and core stability and strength.

starting position

Align yourself correctly in the Relaxation Position. In one controlled, dynamic movement lift your pelvis and spine off the mat so that you can place your hands under the pelvis as support.

Be careful not to place any weight on the head or neck.

Maintain an appropriate level of connection to your centre throughout.

action

● Breathe in and fold one leg in towards the body and then straighten the leg, reaching it directly above the hip. Softly point your foot.

● Breathe out as you flex the foot and lengthen through the back of the leg, to lower the leg down towards the mat. Make sure that your pelvis and spine remain still and stable; lower the leg only as far as this is possible.

● Breathe in, point your foot and swiftly raise the leg back above your hip.

● Repeat this lifting and lowering action three times and then bend the knee back in and return it to the mat.

Repeat three times on the opposite leg.

To finish, once both feet have returned down, roll the spine down to the mat.

WATCH POINTS

★　Maintain stability and stillness in your pelvis throughout. Move your legs independently from your pelvis and spine.

★　Stand firmly into the supporting leg to help keep you grounded and stable.

★　Both the supporting leg and the leg that is moving should remain correctly aligned; i.e. at the hip, knee and ankle.

jack knife

Mobilises the spine, while strengthening the abdominals, hips and legs.

starting position

Align yourself correctly in the Relaxation Position. Connect your inner thighs together and Double Knee Fold both legs in towards you. Straighten both legs directly above your pelvis, turn them out into Pilates Stance and then lower them to a point where you can still maintain a neutral pelvis and spine.
Maintain an appropriate level of connection to your centre throughout.

action

- Breathe in and, with control, begin to draw the legs in towards your body.
- Breathe out and roll your pelvis and then peel the spine one vertebra at a time off the mat. Once your legs are reaching overhead, reach them up and forward above the pelvis.
- Breathe in and begin to roll your spine down onto the mat, wheeling one vertebra at a time. For as long as possible try to keep the legs reaching upwards and try to avoid the legs hinging down towards your face.
- Breathe out, continue to roll through your lower back and, once your pelvis has returned to the mat, reach the legs forwards and lower them to the Starting Position, returning to a neutral pelvis and spine.
Repeat up to five times.
To finish, bend both knees and, keeping the inner thighs connected, lower the legs back down to the mat.

WATCH POINTS

★ To lift into the Jack Knife position, focus on opening the front of the hip joints by gently engaging your inner thighs and buttock muscles.

★ Focus on lifting and lengthening the legs and the pelvis away from the spine in order to avoid any compression.

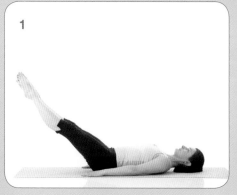

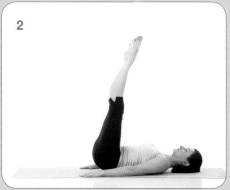

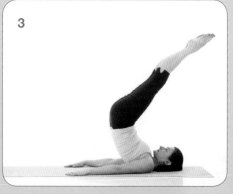

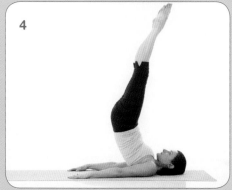

side kick series – side passé

Helps mobilise and strengthen your hips while challenging your spinal stability.

starting position

Lie on your left side, in a straight line, correctly stacking your shoulder, hips and ankles. Carry both legs forward, hinging from the hip joints, so that they are at an angle slightly in front of your body. Your pelvis and spine should remain in neutral.

Prop your head up on your right arm; your elbow is in line with your shoulder. Place your left hand behind your head with your elbow reaching towards the ceiling.

Keeping your pelvis still, turn out your left leg from the hip and softly point your foot. Lengthen your legs and actively connect your inner thighs.

Maintain an appropriate level of connection to your centre throughout.

action

● Breathe in, and keeping your pelvis still, lengthen and lift your left leg directly up. Then, maintaining the turn-out of the leg, bend your knee, bringing your foot to the inside of the underneath knee.

● Breathe out as you slide your foot along the underneath leg, straightening your right leg and reconnecting your inner thighs in the Starting Position.

Repeat three times and then reverse the movement.

● Breathe in and bend your left knee, drawing the foot up the inside of the lower leg. Then, keeping your left thigh still and maintaining the turn-out, straighten your leg, reaching your foot towards the ceiling.

● Breathe out and slowly lower the leg back down to reconnect your inner thighs.

Repeat five times and then either continue with the Side Kick Series on the same side or repeat on the other side.

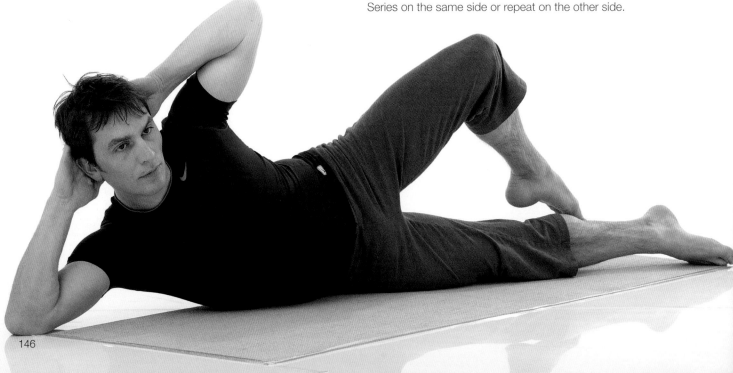

1

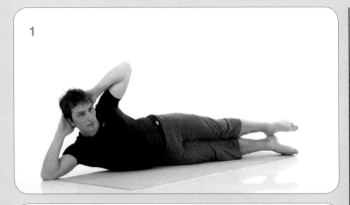

2

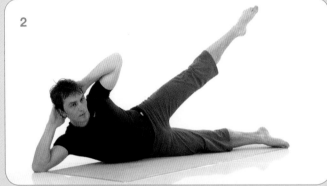

3

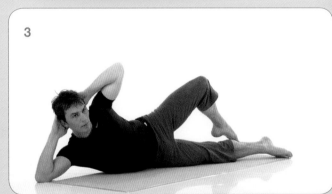

4

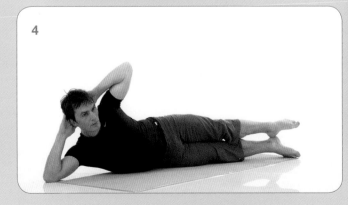

5

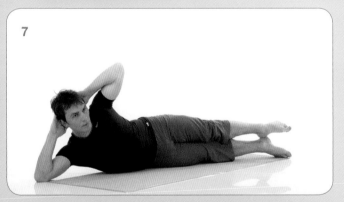

6

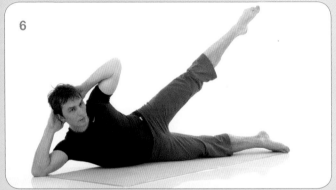

7

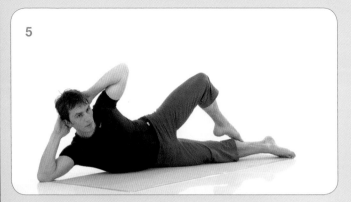

WATCH POINTS

★ Ensure that your pelvis remains stable throughout; move your leg in isolation from the rest your body.

★ Maintain the turn-out of the leg from the hip and not the knee.

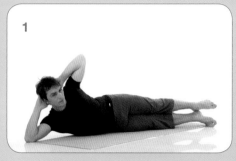

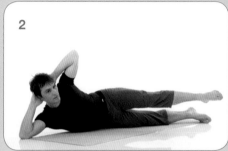

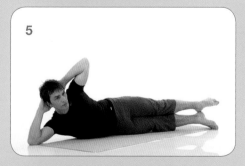

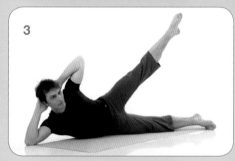

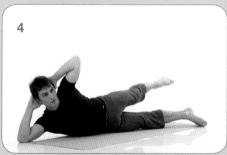

side kick series – big circles

Helps mobilise and strengthen your hips while challenging your spinal stability.

starting position

Lie on your right side and position yourself as for Side Passé (page 146). Maintain an appropriate level of connection to your centre throughout.

action

● Breathe in and, keeping your pelvis still, sweep your left leg forward, hinging from the hip joint. As you reach the end of the sweep forward, begin to lift the leg up and circle it high, above the hip joint.

● Breathe out, continue to circle your leg behind the body and then draw the leg down and circle it around to return to the Starting Position.

Repeat five times and reverse the direction.

● Breathe in and, keeping your pelvis still, reach your left leg behind the body. Then lift and reach it high above the hip joint.

● Breathe out as you circle your leg forwards and down to return to the Starting Position.

Repeat five times. Either continue with the Side Kick Series on the same side or repeat on the other side.

WATCH POINTS

★ Although there will be a slight reactive movement in the pelvis, keep any spinal movement to a minimum.

★ Maintain the turn-out of the leg throughout and ensure that this rotation comes from your hip and not your knee.

side kick series – inner thigh lift

Mobilises and strengthens your hips, with particular focus on the inner thigh muscles, while challenging your spinal stability.

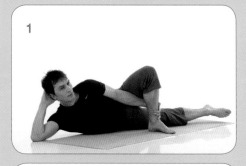

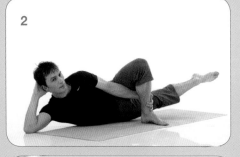

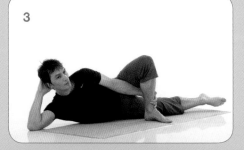

starting position

Lie on your left side and position yourself as for Big Circles (page 148).

Bend your left leg over your right leg and place your foot flat on the mat. Your left heel will be in contact with the centre of your right thigh. Keep the weight on the foot and the knee open to the ceiling.

Wrap your left hand under from the inside of the leg around to the outside of the ankle.

Slightly turn your right leg out from the hip.

Maintain an appropriate level of connection to your centre throughout.

action

● Breathe in as you lengthen and lift the lower leg directly up.

● Breathe out and lower your leg back down with control.

Repeat up to ten times and then either repeat on the other side or begin the entire Side Kick Series on the other side.

(If performing the Advanced Matwork Sequence, you will now have completed the entire Side Kick Series on one side; now perform the Prone Beats (page 122) before turning over onto the other side to repeat the entire Side Kick Series again. Finish off with the Prone Beats to ensure that you are balanced and ready to continue.)

WATCH POINTS

★ Avoid simply resting in the Starting Position, but feel length and energy throughout your entire body.

★ Keep your chest open, and your focus directly ahead of you.

★ Maintain the turn-out of your underneath leg throughout, and ensure that this rotation comes from your hip and not your knee.

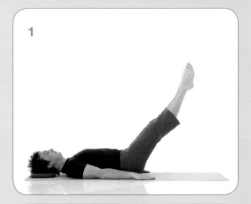

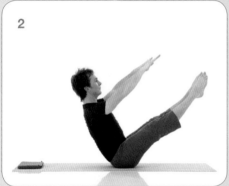

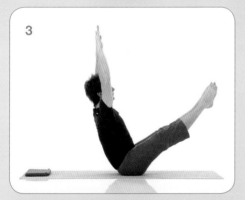

the teaser series

Promotes sequential mobilisation of the spine and is the ultimate in abdominal strengthening, requiring much balance and control.

teaser I

starting position

Align yourself correctly in the Relaxation Position. Connect your inner thighs together and Double Knee Fold both legs in towards you; keeping your heels connected and your feet softly pointed, open your knees slightly.

Breathe in, preparing your body to move, and, as you breathe out, straighten your legs forward on a low diagonal, to a point where you can still maintain a neutral pelvis and spine. Do not allow your lower back to arch. Connect your inner thighs together in Pilates Stance.

Maintain an appropriate level of connection to your centre throughout.

action

● Breathe in as you lengthen the back of your neck, nod your head forwards and sequentially curl your spine off the mat. Maintain the position of your legs until the spine creates a 'V' position with the legs. Your lower back is still slightly rounded but your upper back is lengthened and lifted up. Raise your arms up by the side of your head, focus forwards and open your chest.

● Breathe out as you roll the pelvis underneath you and continue to roll your spine back down onto the mat in a wheeling motion. Lower the arms, returning them by the side of your body – your head will finally return to the mat. Maintain the position of the legs and continue to reach them away on a diagonal line.

Repeat up to five times.

To finish, bend both knees and, keeping the inner thighs connected, lower the legs back down to the mat.

WATCH POINTS

★ Ensure that you wheel smoothly through each segment of your spine.

★ Maintain the length and placement of your legs throughout.

teaser II

starting position

Position yourself as for Teaser I (page 150).
Maintain an appropriate level of connection to your centre throughout.

action

● Breathe in as you lengthen the back of your neck, nod your head forwards and sequentially curl your spine off the mat. Maintain the position of your legs until the spine creates a 'V' position with the legs. Your lower back is still slightly rounded, but your upper back is lengthened and lifted up. Raise your arms up by the side of your head, focus forwards and open your chest.

● Breathe out and lower the legs towards the mat. The movement is small and controlled; the pelvis and spine remain stable.

● Breathe in and draw the legs back in towards the body, returning to the 'V' position.

● Repeat the lift and lower three times. Focus on lengthening the arms and spine up and away from the legs.

● Breathe out, roll the pelvis underneath you and continue to roll your spine back down onto the mat in a wheeling motion. Lower the arms, returning them to the side of your body; your head will finally return to the mat. Maintain the position of the legs, continuing to reach them away on a diagonal line.
Repeat up to five times.

To finish, bend both knees and, keeping the inner thighs connected, lower the legs back down to the mat.

WATCH POINTS

★　Lower the legs as far towards the mat as possible whilst maintaining a strong core connection and a stable and still pelvis and spine.

★　As your legs lower, reach continuously upwards with the arms and your upper spine – encourage a sense of lift and opposition.

★　Lower the legs slowly and with control as you exhale and lift them briskly back up as you inhale.

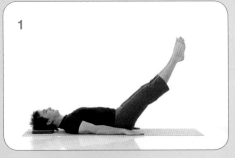

1

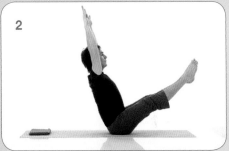

2

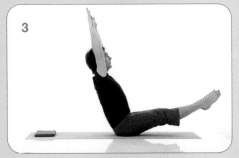

3

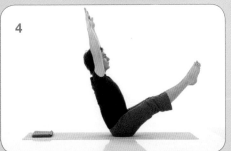

4

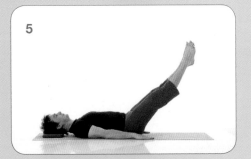

5

teaser III

starting position

Lie on your back with both legs straight, and your inner thighs connected in Pilates Stance. Softly point your feet. Your pelvis and spine are in neutral. Raise your arms overhead with your palms facing up and maintain openness across the chest. Maintain an appropriate level of connection to your centre throughout.

This is the ultimate of the Teaser Series and requires you to roll the spine and lift the legs simultaneously without momentum.

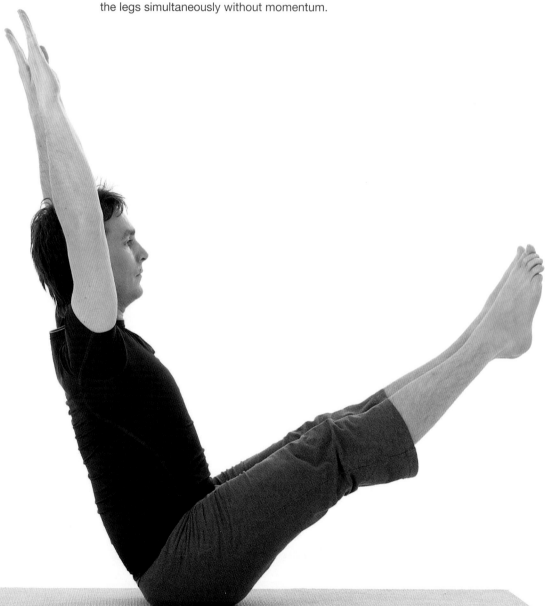

action

● Breathe in as you raise your arms and nod your head forwards, and sequentially curl your spine off the mat. Simultaneously lengthen and lift both legs off the mat to meet your spine in the 'V' position. Throughout the roll your arms remain overhead. Focus forwards and open your chest.

● Breathe out, roll the pelvis underneath you and continue to roll your spine back down onto the mat in a wheeling motion. At the same time, lower your legs to the mat, controlling and coordinating the movement with your spine. Once again the arms remain lengthened overhead.

Repeat up to five times.

To finish, bend both knees and, keeping the inner thighs connected, lower the legs back down to the mat.

WATCH POINTS

★ Ensure a smooth and sequential roll through the spine. It is particularly easy, when lifting the legs, to merely hinge the spine up.

★ Coordinate the correct timing of the legs and the spine lowering and lifting.

★ Ensure that you wheel smoothly through each segment of your spine, on the roll up as well as on the roll down.

★ Roll directly through your centre line avoiding any deviations to either side.

★ Fully straighten your legs but avoid locking your knees.

★ Keep a relationship between the shoulders and the back of your ribcage. Neither force them to depress, nor allow them to over-elevate.

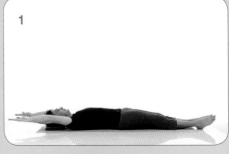

1

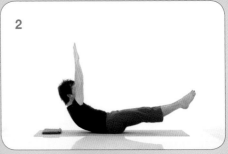

2

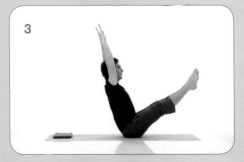

3

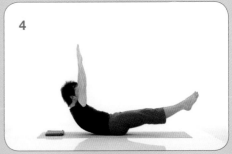

4

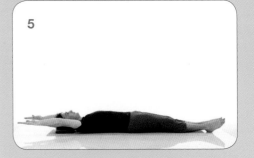

5

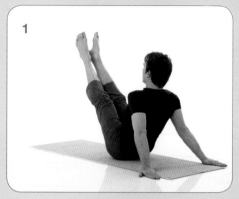

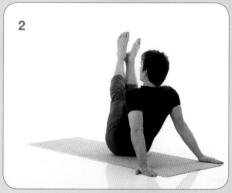

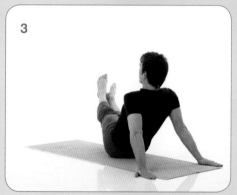

hip circles

Develop strength and stamina in the abdominal and hip area while mobilising the lower back.

starting position

Sit upright with legs bent in front of you, feet on the mat. Straighten your arms and circle them behind your body to place the palms on the mat, fingers facing away from you. Your pelvis is rolled underneath you so that you can balance on the back of your pelvis (not your sitting bones). Your upper spine is lengthened and lifted, your focus is forwards and your chest is open.

Breathe in, preparing your body to move, and, as you breathe out, maintaining a strong and stable centre, straighten your legs and lift your feet off the mat to create a 'V' position with your spine and your legs. Connect your inner thighs in Pilates Stance and softly point your feet.

Maintain an appropriate level of connection to your centre throughout.

The movement is continuous, flowing and dynamic without momentum.

action

● Breathe in and reach the legs to the right, allowing your pelvis to roll. The left side of the pelvis will slightly roll away from the mat but your ribcage, chest and head must remain square to the front.

● Breathe out, lower the legs and circle them to arrive at the centre line of the body. Your pelvis must still be rolled underneath; use your deep abdominals to prevent the weight of the legs pulling the pelvis and arching the lower back.

● Continue to breathe out and circle the legs and your pelvis to the left, and draw them back up and around to the Starting Position in the centre line.

● Reverse the direction.

Repeat up to five times, reversing the direction of the circle each time.

To finish, bend both knees and, keeping the inner thighs connected, lower the legs back down to the mat.

WATCH POINTS

★ Stay very connected in your deep core muscles throughout; it is essential that your abdominals prevent your spine from arching.

★ Keep your chest open and your upper spine lifted throughout. Maintain the connection of the ribcage to the pelvis and avoid flaring the ribcage.

★ Although the pelvis will roll side to the side, remain long either side of your waist and avoid 'hitching' your pelvis up towards your ribcage.

★ Keep the inner thighs connected and lengthen the legs throughout, but do avoid locking the knees.

★ Control the exercise with a controlled and yet dynamic pace. Use the breathing pattern to help the flow of the movement.

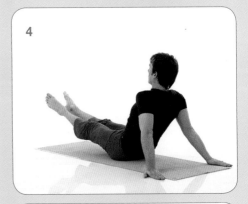

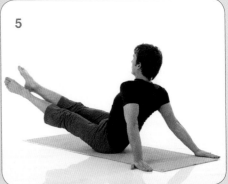

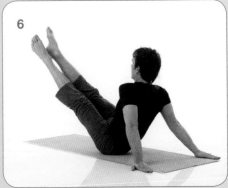

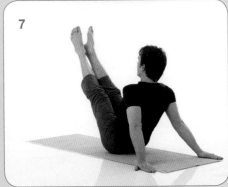

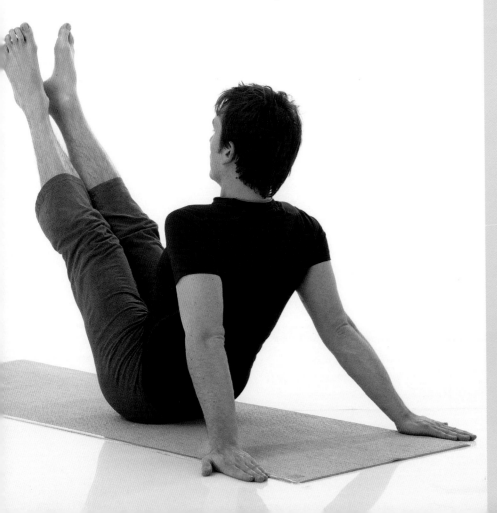

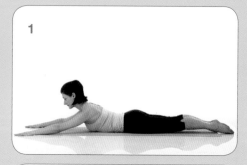

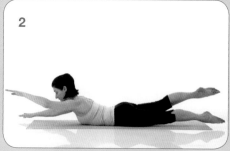

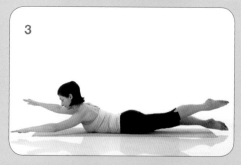

swimming

Promotes spinal stability by moving the arms and legs independently from the torso; also develops strength and stamina in the upper back and shoulder muscles.

starting position

Lie on your front, correctly aligning your pelvis and spine in neutral, and rest your forehead on the mat. Your legs are straight, and the inner thighs connected in parallel. Reach both arms above your head, slightly wider than shoulder width apart and resting on the mat. Your palms are facing down. Lift your head and chest slightly off the mat to extend your upper spine, and look forwards without shortening the back of your neck.

Breathe in, preparing your body to move, and, as you breathe out, maintain a stable torso and lengthen and lift one arm off the mat and, at the same time, slightly raise the opposite leg.

Maintain an appropriate level of connection to your centre throughout.

Your goal is to maintain a lengthened spine and a stable core while you beat the arms and the legs freely and dynamically. Although the pace of the exercise is fairly fast, it should not be frantic.

action

● Breathe in for a count of five as you lower and lift the opposite arms and legs in a light beating motion. Relate the movement to the breathing pattern and switch the arms and legs five times.

● Breathe out for a count of five and once again exchange the opposite arms and legs in a swimming motion.

Repeat five times.

To finish, release your head and spine and lower your arms and legs back down to the mat. Press up onto your hands and knees and then fold back into the Rest Position (page 28) to allow your spine to release.

WATCH POINTS

★ Ensure that there is no compression or shortening of your lower spine. Keep your abdominals connected but allow them to lengthen fully without collapse.

★ Keep the legs straight as they beat and focus on the front of your hips opening. You will feel the backs of the legs and the buttocks working to lift the legs. Your pelvis should remain grounded and still.

kneeling side kicks

Mobilise and strengthen your hips while challenging your spinal stability and balance.

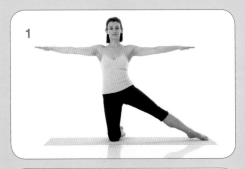

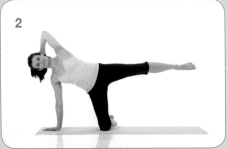

starting position

Kneel upright. Raise both arms out to the side at shoulder height, palms facing down. Lengthen your left leg directly out to the side in line with your pelvis and softly point your foot. Breathe in, preparing your body to move, and, as you breathe out, lengthen your waist and lean to the right, raising the left leg off the mat and placing your right hand on the mat. The right arm is straight and supportive; the left leg is also straight, reaching directly in line with the pelvis and parallel to the mat. Bend your left arm and place the hand behind your head.
Maintain an appropriate level of connection to your centre throughout.

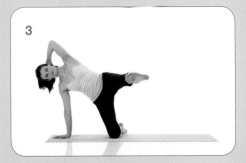

action

● Breathe in and, maintaining a strong and stable centre, swing the left leg forwards, ensuring that you keep your torso long and still.
● Breathe out and carry the left leg back again, reaching it slightly behind the pelvis but not so far that you arch your back or push your torso forwards.
Repeat five kicks with the left leg and then repeat, balancing on the other side.
To finish, lower your leg to the mat and lift your torso back to the vertical Starting Position, your arms returning lengthened at shoulder height.

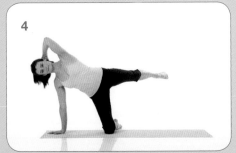

WATCH POINTS

★   Keep your supporting leg still and open in the front of the hip.

★   The quality of the movement should be brisk and yet controlled.

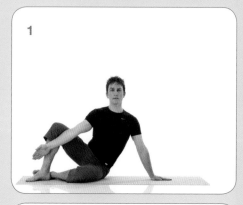

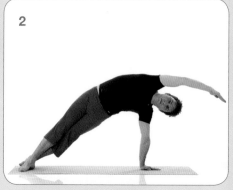

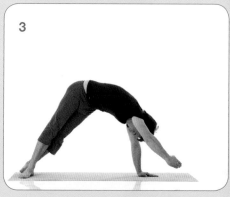

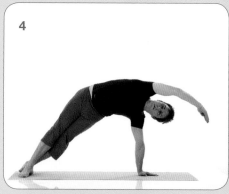

side twist

Mobilises the spine and develops shoulder strength and stability while creating openness in the chest and the front of the shoulders.

starting position

Sit on your left hip with the left leg bent underneath you. The foot is in line with your pelvis.

With your left arm supporting you, place the left palm on the mat, outstretched directly to the side. Cross your right foot over the left ankle so that the sole of the foot is flat on the mat in preparation to take your weight. Turn out the right leg from the hip, so that the right knee is lifted up to the ceiling. Your pelvis is lifted as upright as possible and square to the front.

Maintain an appropriate level of connection to your centre throughout.

action

● Breathe in as you begin to lift the pelvis and circle your right arm overhead, simultaneously straighten your legs, connecting your inner thighs. Reach over to the left in a high arc, stretching the spine and the legs.

● Breathe out as you turn your head, chest and ribs towards the mat; stay lifted. Keep the right arm by your head as you feel your spine curling inwards. Allow the pelvis to twist slightly and rise. Deepen the connection of your abdominals.

● Breathe in as you continue to lengthen the spine and twist back to return squarely to the centre. Raise the right arm above your shoulder, lengthening up towards the ceiling.

● Still breathing in, turn your head and chest towards the ceiling and allow your right arm to open slightly to the right. Keep the legs tightly connected and do not allow the pelvis or lower back to move.

● Breathe out as you return the head, chest and arm to the centre before bending the knees, circling the right arm down and returning to the Starting Position on the mat.

Repeat up to five times and then repeat on the other side.

WATCH POINTS

★ During the initial side stretch try to maintain the torso and legs square to the front.

★ As the spine twists around towards the mat it should be a spiralling action, i.e. beginning with the arms and then the head and then coiling into the chest and ribcage and finally into the abdominal area which should be very connected and lifted.

★ Remain lifted away from the supporting arm at all times and do not allow the elbow to lock.

★ The top arm should always move in response to the position of the upper spine. It is the spine that initiates all of the movement and not the arm swinging around.

★ Keep your inner thighs connected as the legs straighten. Avoid locking your knees.

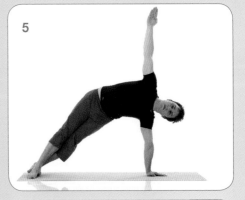

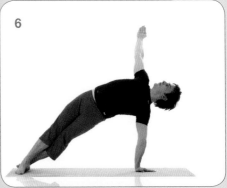

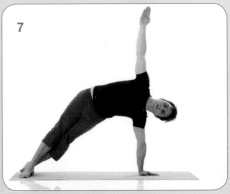

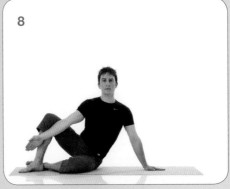

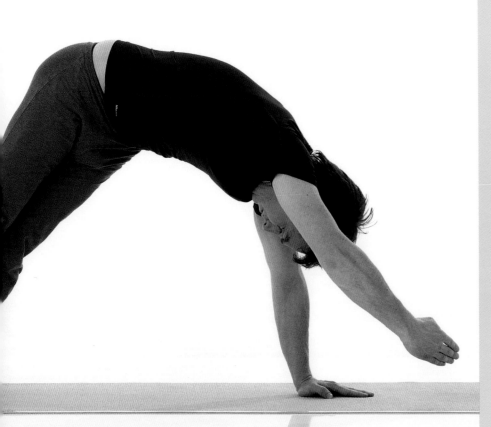

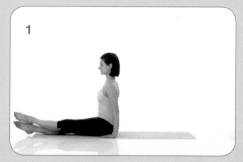

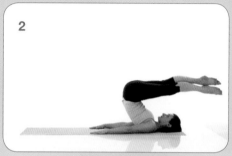

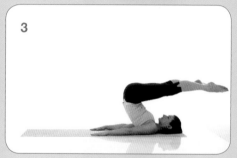

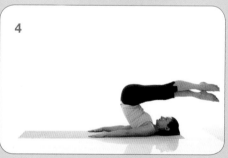

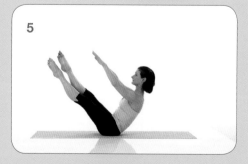

boomerang

Focuses on the strength and mobility of the spine, legs and shoulders, fully incorporating balance, control and precision.

starting position

Sit upright with your legs lengthened out in front of your body. Your pelvis and spine are in neutral. Turn your legs out slightly and cross one leg over the other. Your arms are lengthening down by your sides and your palms are placed on the mat next to the pelvis.

Maintain an appropriate level of connection to your centre throughout.

Enjoy the continuous flow of the sequence. Control the exercise with a precise yet dynamic pace, using the breathing pattern to help the flow of the movement.

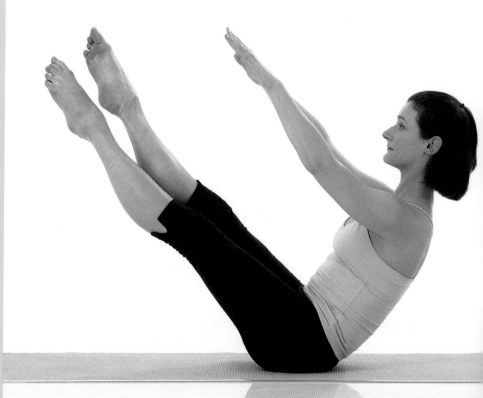

action

- Breathe in, preparing your body to move, and lengthen your spine.
- Breathe out as you press your hands down into the mat and roll the spine backwards, lifting the legs almost immediately. Roll the spine off the mat to the tips of the shoulder blades. The legs should now be folded over the torso and parallel to the mat.
- Breathe in, open your legs shoulder-width apart and close them, this time crossing the other leg on top.
- Breathe out. Keeping the relationship between the legs and the spine, roll back up to balance on the back of the pelvis with the legs reaching forwards on a high diagonal and the arms reaching straight ahead at shoulder-height. Keep your pelvis curled underneath you so that you are balancing on the back of your pelvis and not on your sitting bones.
- Breathe in as you circle your arms behind you. Clasp the hands behind your body and straighten the arms, pressing them further behind you. Open the front of the shoulders and lift the chest.
- Breathe out and with control lower the legs to the mat and fold the spine up and over the legs. Keep the hands clasped and press your arms upwards and away from your spine.
- Breath in, release your hands and circle the arms up and around and finally over and towards the feet.
- Breathe out. Initiating from your centre, roll the spine up to vertical, re-stacking one vertebra at a time. Return your arms to the sides of your pelvis, palms flat down into the mat.

Repeat up to six times.

WATCH POINTS

★ Maintain length in your spine throughout and feel constant support from the abdominals.

★ Use your arms pressing down to help with the initial roll back when lifting your legs, but do not use momentum.

★ Focus on lifting and lengthening the legs and the pelvis away from the spine in order to avoid any compression.

★ Open and close the legs briskly to reconnect the inner thighs.

★ When in the 'V' position, keep the chest open and your upper spine lifted but avoid flaring the ribcage.

6
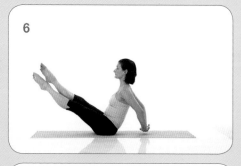

7
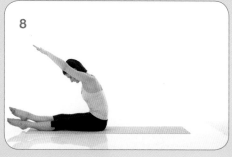

8
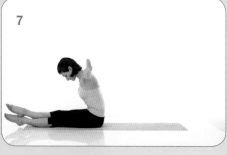

9
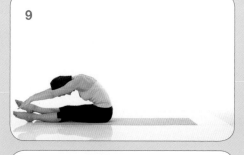

10
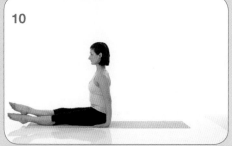

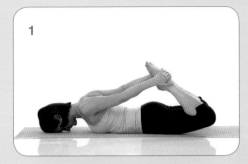

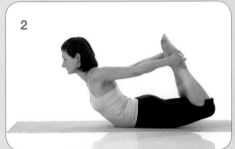

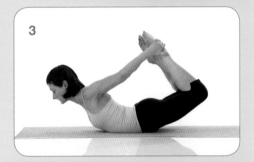

rocking

Develops strength and stamina in the muscles in the back of the spine, hips and legs while lengthening and opening the front of the body.

starting position

Lie on your front and rest your forehead on the mat. Bend your knees, drawing your heels towards your buttocks. Reach the arms behind you and take hold of the ankles. The knees will be hip-width apart or slightly wider.

Breathe in as you press the ankles into your hands. Actively engage your buttocks and the backs of your legs. Begin to lift your head, chest and, if possible, ribcage off the mat, creating an extended, arched and lengthened spine.

Maintain an appropriate level of connection to your centre throughout.

The goal of this exercise is to find the lengthened and arched shape of the legs and spine and maintain this position as you rock forwards and back.

This action requires a strong spine and a lot of breath control.

action

● Breathe out, maintaining the arched shape of the spine and the legs as you rock forwards. Roll onto your chest area, reaching the feet even further up and behind you.

● Breathe in as you maintain the established arc position and press the ankles into your hands to rock back up. Lift your head and chest as you rock onto the fronts of your thighs.

Repeat up to five times.

To finish, release your legs and return your head, spine, legs and arms to the mat. Then press up onto your hands and knees and fold back into the Rest Position (page 28) to allow your spine to release.

Advice: Never force the body to rock. To begin with, merely find the Starting Position and lift the body away from the mat as you inhale and return back down to the Starting Position as you exhale.

WATCH POINTS

★ Ensure that there is no compression or shortening of your lower spine. Keep your abdominals connected but allow them to lengthen fully without collapse.

★ Emphasise the pressing-up of the legs during the rock forwards and the pressing-away of the legs during the rock up.

control and balance

As well as developing control and balance, this exercise also lengthens the back of the spine and the legs, while challenging stability and developing core strength.

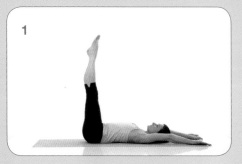

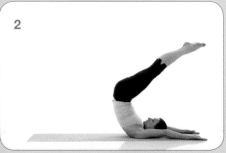

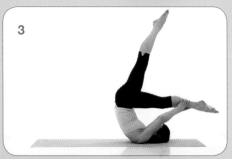

starting position

Align yourself correctly in the Relaxation Position. Connect your inner thighs together and Double Knee Fold both legs in towards you. Straighten both legs directly above your pelvis and softly point your feet.

Raise both arms overhead, lengthening them along the mat with the palms facing the ceiling.

Breathe in, preparing your body to move, and, as you breathe out, with control, draw the legs in towards your body and roll your pelvis and then peel the spine one vertebra at a time off the mat. Maintaining balance and control, reach your legs up to the ceiling in a Jack-knife position.

Maintain an appropriate level of connection to your centre throughout.

action

● Breathe in as you lower the right leg overhead, keeping it straight; before it reaches the mat take hold of the ankle and lengthen. Simultaneously reach the left leg directly up to the ceiling, achieving a vertical stretch.

● Breathe out and, controlling the balance of the position, exchange the legs, reaching the right toward the ceiling and lowering and holding the left leg to lengthen it behind your head.

Repeat this exchange up to six times.

To finish, connect the legs, reaching them upwards, and sequentially roll the spine back down. Then lower the legs, returning to the Relaxation Position.

WATCH POINTS

★ From your centre, focus on lifting and lengthening the legs and the pelvis away from the spine in order to avoid any compression.

★ Avoid rolling too far over. The weight should be across the upper back, not the head and neck.

★ As the legs switch, ensure that the exchange takes place approximately halfway through the full range of movement of the legs.

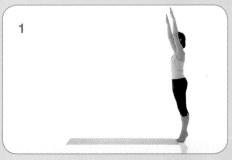

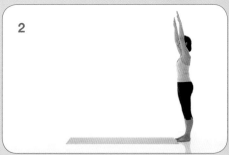

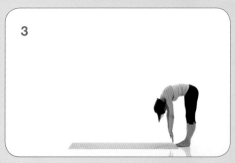

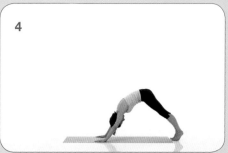

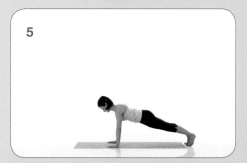

press up

Develops not only strength and stability in the shoulders and arms, but also requires a great deal of power in the core.

starting position

Stand tall on the floor (not on your mat) and lengthen your spine into neutral. Connect your inner thighs in Pilates Stance and raise your arms directly above your head, palms facing forwards. Maintain the connection of the inner thighs and your heels and rise up onto the balls of the feet.

Maintain an appropriate level of connection to your centre throughout.

Use this exercise to consolidate all that you have learnt and achieved in the Advanced Matwork Programme. Finish in the standing position feeling entirely grounded, lengthened and strengthened.

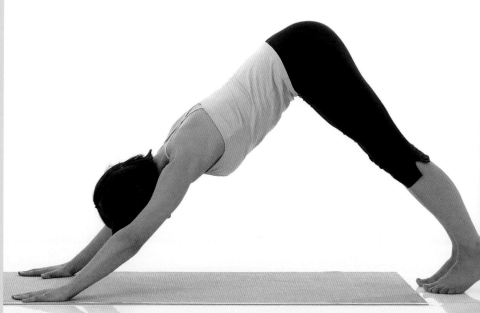

action

- Breathe in, preparing your body to move, and lengthen your spine.
- Breathe out as you lower your heels to the mat, maintaining length and opposition in the arms and the spine.
- Breathe in as you lower your arms and nod your head to begin sequentially rolling your spine forwards and down, until the hands reach the mat.
- Breathe out and begin to walk the hands out in front of you. Keep the heels pressing into the mat. When the heels have to lift, lengthen the spine out into a Plank position. Your wrists should be directly underneath your shoulders and the pelvis and spine in a lengthened and supported neutral position.
- Breathe in; bend your elbows, keeping them in close to your body. Your entire body will lower towards the mat and you must remain strong and stable in your centre.
- Breathe out and straighten your elbows, pressing the body back up.
- Repeat this Press Up three times.
- Breathe in; from your hips fold your torso back towards the legs, creating an inverted 'V' position. Press the heels down into the mat once again.
- Breathe out as you begin to walk the hands back in towards the feet, folding your torso towards your legs.
- Breathe in, curling your pelvis underneath and then roll up to the vertical position, re-stacking your spine vertebra by vertebra. Once you have returned upright, rise up onto the balls of your feet and raise your arms overhead. Repeat three times.

WATCH POINTS

★ As you initially roll down, ensure that you roll smoothly and sequentially through each segment of your spine.

★ Roll directly through your centre line, avoiding any deviations to either side.

★ During the Press Up it is essential to maintain a good abdominal connection to avoid your pelvis and spine dipping down towards the mat.

★ As you straighten your arms, avoid locking your elbows.

★ Maintain a firm connection of the shoulder blades to the back of your ribcage. Even when bending your elbows, focus on the opposition of your body away from your arms and keep your chest open.

6
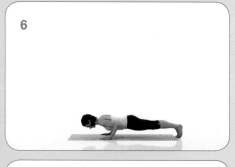

7
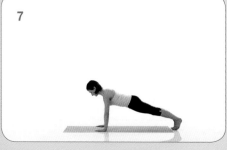

8
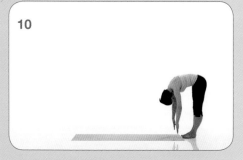

9
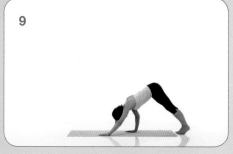

10
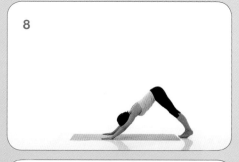

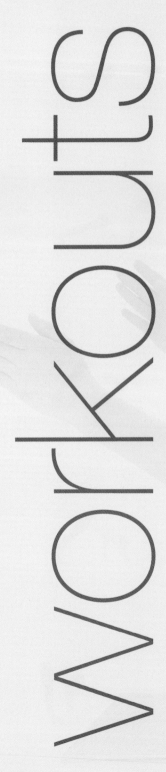

workouts

The Advanced Matwork Sequence

The foundation of the method that Joseph Pilates created was 'The Matwork', a series of over forty exercises that were performed without the use of apparatus.

What follows is our interpretation of his classical work that we will refer to as the Advanced Matwork. As these are the most challenging of all Pilates exercises we advise that you do not attempt the sequence until you have mastered the fundamental principles of the Beginners' and Intermediate Programmes.

Before embarking on the Advanced Matwork, it is a good idea to do a full body awareness 'warm up' using exercises from the Beginners' Programme. Use the exercises to help pattern movements and to enable your mind to focus on your body and your breath.

Although it may well take you time to master each exercise individually, remember that your ultimate goal is to link all of the exercises together to create a flowing sequence. Respect the order that the exercises have been placed in – it is understandable if you feel the need to omit certain exercises, but otherwise continue to pattern the exercises in the intended order. When placed within the carefully selected structure, each exercise will take on more meaning.

The order has been structured to allow the body to experience a balance of movement encompassing all planes, utilising all joints and muscles and equalising strength with mobility. The sequence develops in a progressive manner, allowing you to challenge your body gradually and effectively.

We have deliberately not specified how to move from one exercise to the next (transition). We will leave this up to you. Just remember that during each transition you should remain 'in the moment', staying focused on your breath, your alignment and your centre. This will help you to move more efficiently and with precision. Through this integration of seamless movement you will find the whole experience invigorating and challenging.

1. The Hundred
2. Roll Up
3. Roll Over
4. Leg Circles
5. Rolling Like a Ball
6. Single Leg Stretch
7. Double Leg Stretch
8. Single Straight Leg Stretch
9. Double Straight Leg Raises
10. Criss-cross
11. Spine Stretch Forward
12. Open Leg Rocker
13. Corkscrew
14. The Saw
15. Swan Dive
16. Single Leg Kick
17. Double Leg Kick
18. Neck Pull
19. Scissors
20. Bicycle
21. Shoulder Bridge
22. Spine Twist
23. Jack-knife
24. Side Kick Series – Front and Back
25. Side Kick Series – Up and Down
26. Side Kick Series – Small Circles
27. Side Kick Series – Side Passé
28. Side Kick Series – Big Circles
29. Side Kick Series – Inner Thigh Lift
30. Prone Beats
31. Teaser I
32. Teaser II
33. Teaser III
34. Hip Circles
35. Swimming
36. Leg Pull Front
37. Leg Pull Back
38. Kneeling Side Kicks
39. Side Twist
40. Boomerang
41. Seal
42. Rocking
43. Control and Balance
44. Press Up

Chapter Five:
Pilates Equipment

Studio equipment adds another dimension to the Pilates method, providing many benefits that serve to enhance the effectiveness of the matwork exercises. In this section we introduce you to the four most commonly used pieces of equipment along with images that demonstrate just some of the wonderful exercise possibilities they offer. For safety and effectiveness we recommend that you use studio equipment under the guidance of a qualified teacher (see Further Information, page 284).

The magic of working with studio equipment is the additional benefits it offers over working with matwork exercises alone. Machines like the Reformer, Cadillac and Chair provide variable resistance via springs that can be used to improve strength and control or to provide a level of assistance that allows you to attempt movements and positions that would otherwise be impossible. The moving parts of these machines also facilitate flowing movements with control, challenging stability in one direction while providing stability and control in another. Equipment like the Barrels provide raised and curved surfaces which can be used to challenge ranges of movement as well as to offer support and feedback throughout the exercises performed on them.

The reformer

The Pilates Reformer is the most popular piece of Pilates studio equipment. Created in the 1920s by Joseph Pilates, the 'Universal Reformer' today remains fundamentally unchanged in terms of design and function.

It is an extremely versatile, resistance-based machine that consists of a complex set of springs, ropes and straps, all connected to a gliding carriage. Exercises can be performed lying down, sitting, kneeling or standing on the carriage and the straps are used to place either your feet or hands in to allow you to push or pull yourself on the carriage against the resistance provided by the springs and your own body weight. The variable tension in the springs allows you to alter resistance according to your own skill level and exercise objectives.

There are simply hundreds of exercises that can be performed on the Reformer, ranging from the fundamentals that can help to consolidate your Beginners' Matwork to extremely advanced work that can challenge you and also help you to prepare for the Advanced Matwork.

footwork

Although it is named Footwork, this series of exercises does, in fact, work the entire body and, as it is performed in a comfortable non-weight-bearing position, it is a great introduction to all of the Pilates principles. Think of Leg Slides, Knee Folds and Tennis Ball Rising in the Beginners' Matwork.

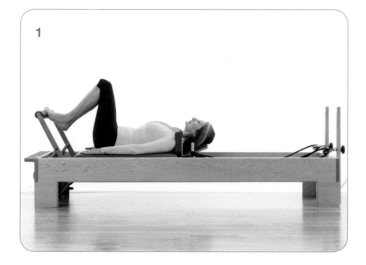

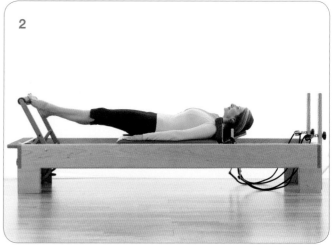

the hundred

This exercise is a great example of how we can challenge an Intermediate Matwork exercise with the instability and added resistance of the Reformer. The ropes also provide sensory feedback to the hands and arms, increasing your awareness of your movement and your position in space.

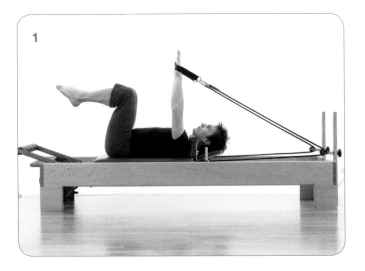

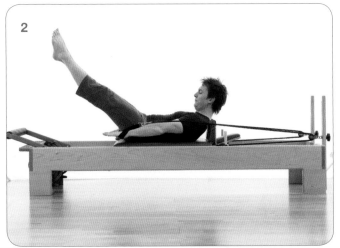

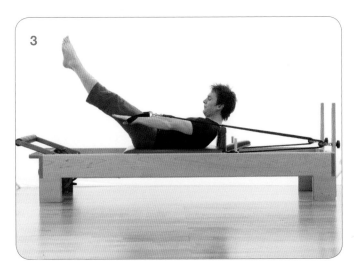

short spine massage

This is a great example of how to modify Advanced Matwork moves such as Roll Over, Corkscrew and Jack Knife by offering the body support to find the ultimate position. Although Short Spine Massage doesn't exactly replicate these mat exercises, the initial spine roll movement is very similar and therefore can be patterned and learned to help gain strength and develop an understanding of the requirements before attempting it on the mat.

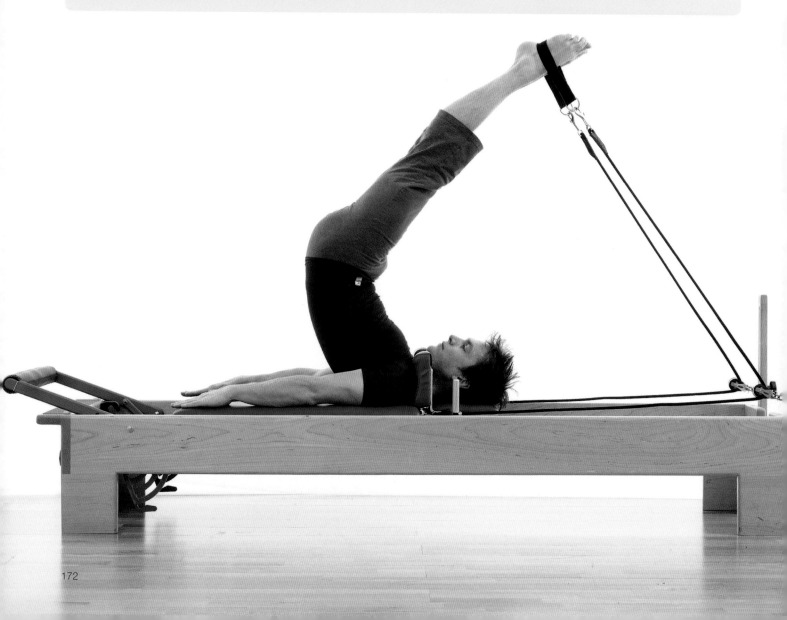

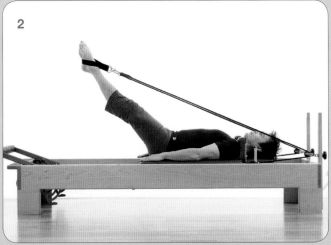

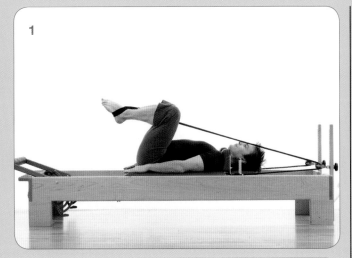

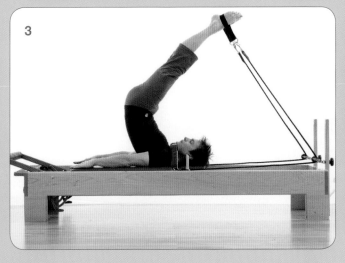

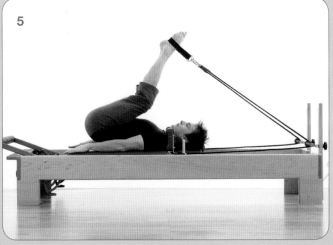

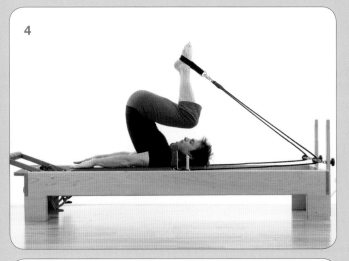

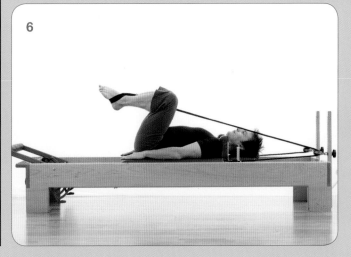

pulling ropes

Pulling Ropes has a similar movement pattern to the Dart but, as a result of the increased flexion in your spine over the box in the Starting Position, you can achieve much more range of movement in your upper back than you would be able to on the mat.

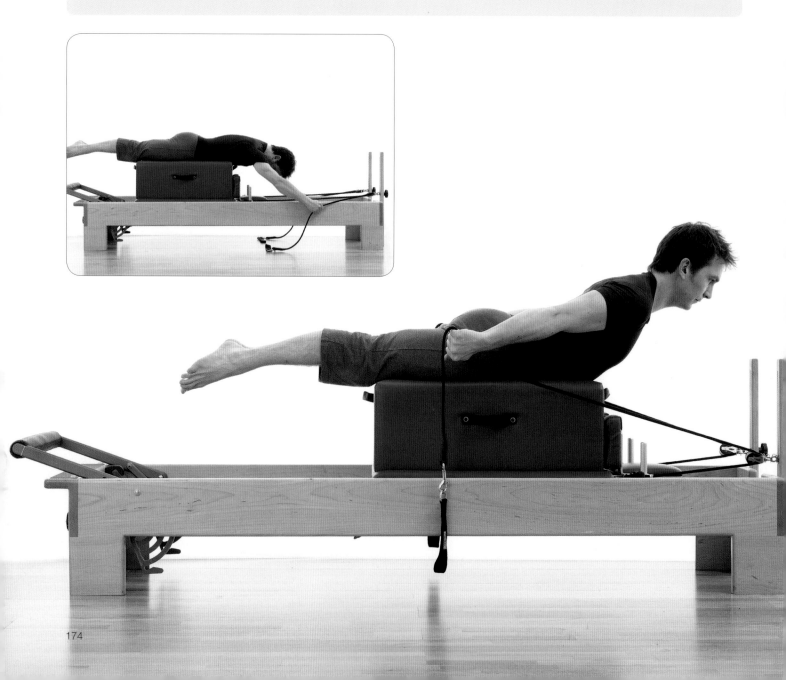

long stretch

Similar to the Press Up in the Advanced Matwork, this exercise challenges the stability of the spine and the shoulder girdle, and the added movement of the carriage offers a sense of length and direction.

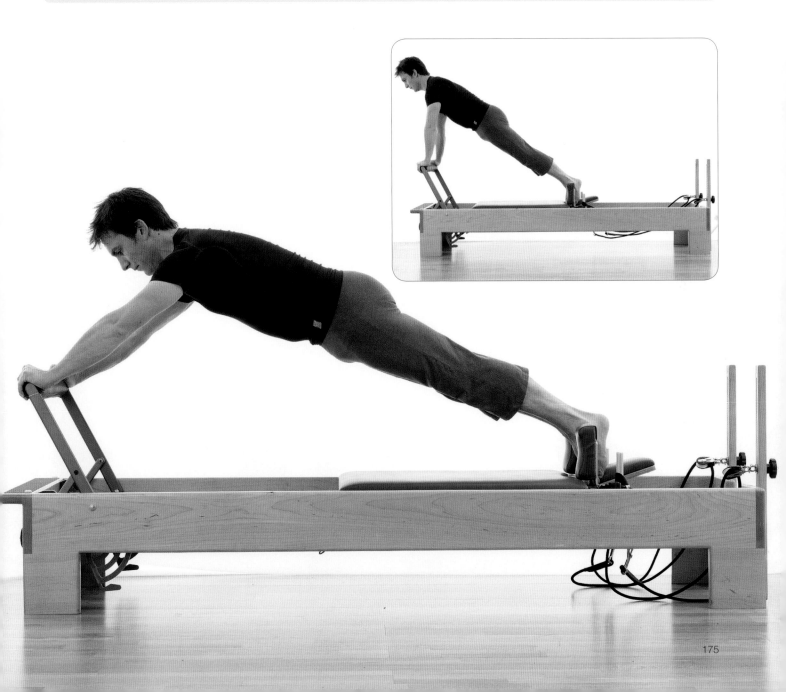

snake

This is a true exercise of full body integration, a classic Pilates exercise that requires every inch of you to be alert and working. It is similar in shape and pattern to the Advanced Matwork exercise Side Twist, but far more challenging.

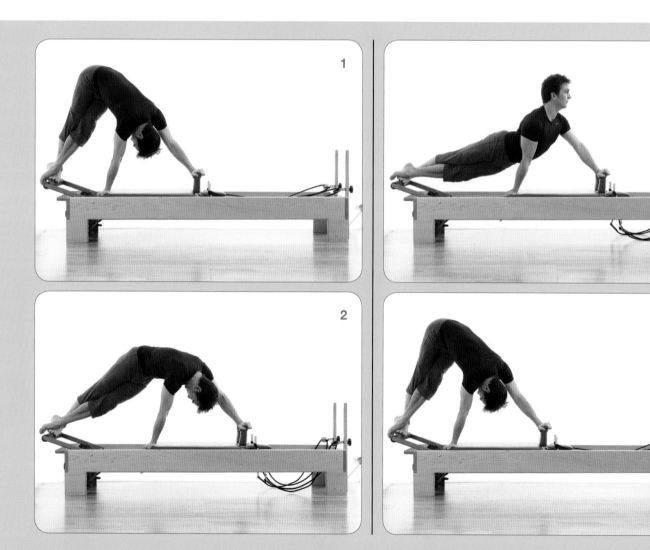

side splits – the saw

As this exercise is performed standing on the Reformer it is an excellent functional challenge for the body in terms of stability, balance and alignment and is very relevant to the awareness of our posture in everyday life. The Saw is an advanced variation of Side Splits, incorporating leg strength and hip mobility with flexion and rotation of the spine.

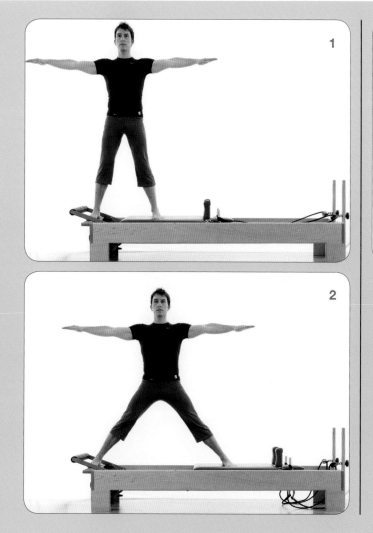

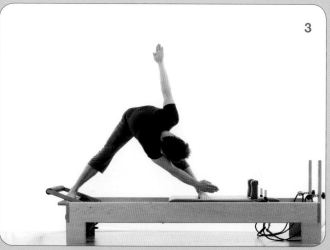

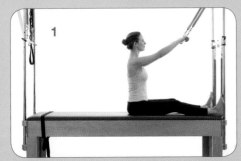

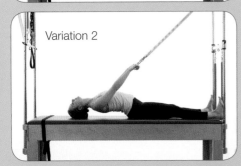

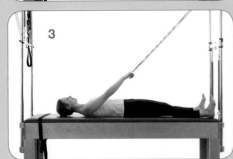

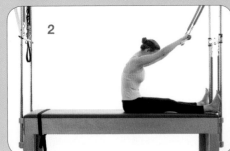

Variation 1

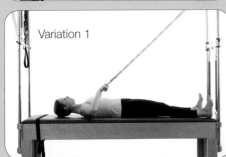

Variation 2

The cadillac

The Cadillac (also known as the Trapeze Table) is another effective and versatile piece of Pilates studio equipment developed by Joseph Pilates. During the First World War, he was working as an orderly in a hospital in an internment camp on the Isle of Man. He helped with rehabilitating patients who were recovering from the flu pandemic and wartime injuries. Wishing to keep his bed-ridden patients mobile and strong, he devised the beginnings of what is now known as the Cadillac by attaching springs to the posts of the bed, thereby allowing patients to exercise with the help of resistance while still in bed.

Of course, the Cadillac has evolved considerably since, but the essence of Joseph's original intentions remains. It consists of various adjustable moving parts and provides resistance through springs in much the same way as the Reformer. These are all attached to a frame and bench that resembles a four-poster bed.

A variety of exercises can be performed on the Cadillac ranging from the basic fundamental principles of the matwork to acrobatic style choreographed sequences. The Cadillac is, therefore, an ideal piece of equipment to suit every level of ability.

roll back

Many people struggle to find the strength and mobility to perform matwork Roll Ups, but with the assistance of the Cadillac springs this exercise can be a smooth and enjoyable way of articulating the spine. Even if you have mastered the Roll Up with no difficulty, the Roll Back on the Cadillac is still an effective and worthwhile exercise.

shoulder roll

This exercise reflects the spinal articulation of such matwork exercises as Roll Over and Jack Knife and also the Short Spine Massage performed on the Reformer. This time the body is working against resistance, so a great deal of focus must be placed on the length and openness in the spine to avoid any compression.

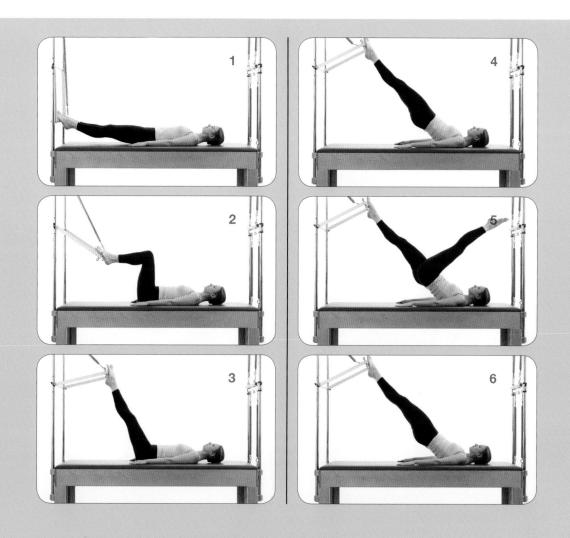

the cat

This is another great example of how we can challenge a Beginners' Matwork exercise by using studio equipment. The added resistance of the springs will work to improve your strength and help you to connect into your centre.

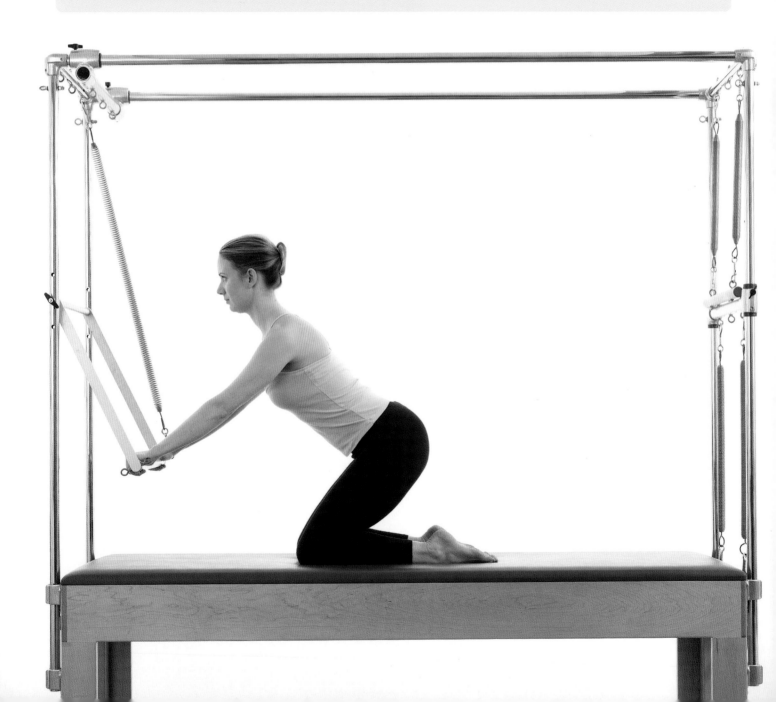

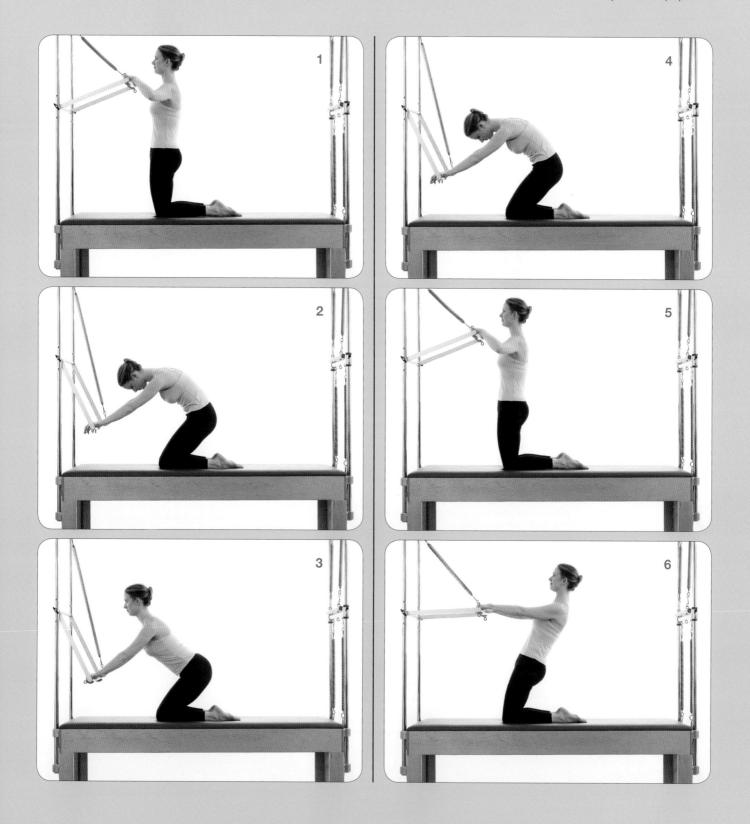

leg springs series – side-lying up and down

The movement of this exercise is exactly the same as the Side Kick Series – Up and Down that you will find in the Intermediate Matwork workout. You are now faced with the added challenge of working against the resistance of the springs, but you will also find the added benefit of working with the springs and discover a slightly bigger range of movement.

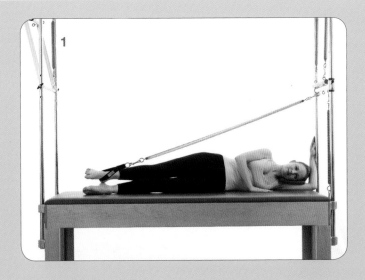

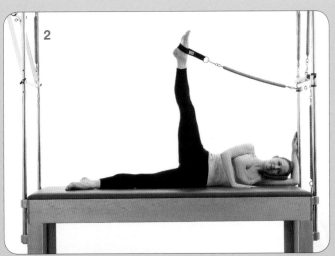

pull ups

This is one of the most impressive, acrobatic exercises in the Pilates repertoire. It is challenging but as long as you have substantial upper body strength, it feels great. The ability to articulate the spine, which you have developed through your Pilates practice, enables you to enjoy the freedom of hanging from the frame like a child in a playground!

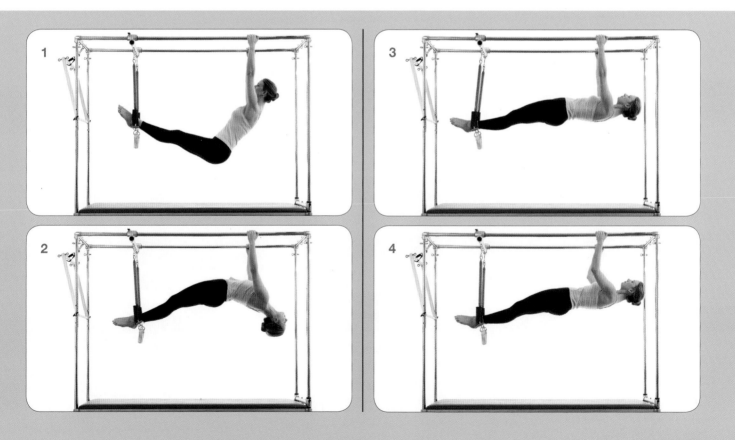

The chair

As with the Reformer and the Cadillac, the Chair helps to build strength and flexibility with adjustable spring resistance. What sets it apart is its size, which adds a new dimension to a Pilates Studio workout. As it is much more compact it provides only a very narrow base of support, thereby considerably increasing the physical and technical challenge of the exercises performed. It's a great piece of equipment for working out in the comfort of your own home, exactly in line with Joseph Pilates' original vision when developing it.

Don't be fooled, though – just because it is called a Chair it does not mean you will be sitting down to do your exercises. The Chair challenges your stability, balance and control in many positions such as standing, kneeling and lying and requires considerable mind-body focus, patience and concentration. Basic functional exercises focusing on posture, mobility and alignment can also be performed by beginners.

There are many variations of the original Chair, including the Wunda Chair, High Chair and Combo Chair. They all fundamentally follow the same design and intention with slight variations based on the exercises taught on them.

footwork

This series of exercises is similar to the Footwork that is performed on the Reformer. However, here we perform the entire series sitting upright, which challenges your upright posture and is effective in improving and strengthening your core stability.

Flat back

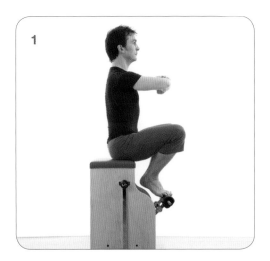
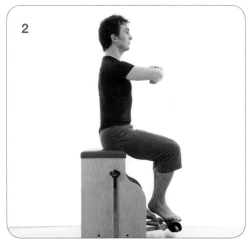

Round back

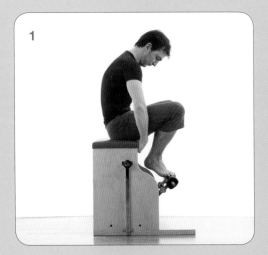
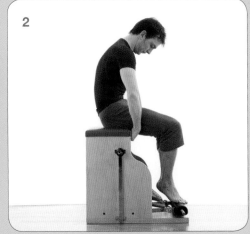

Twist

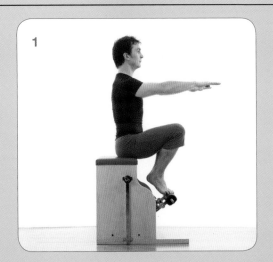
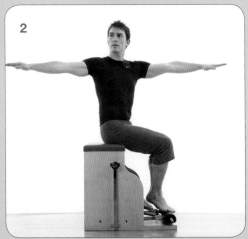

Frog

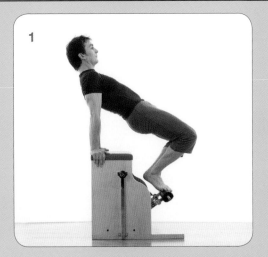
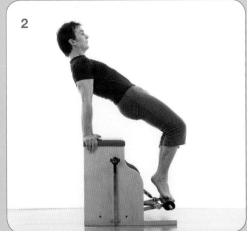

side lifts

This exercise reflects the alignment of Torpedo but, instead of challenging your core by lifting the legs, the Chair allows you the dimensions and support to lift and lower the upper body while keeping the pelvis and legs still.

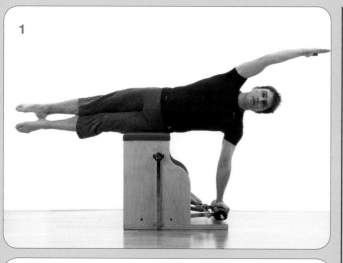

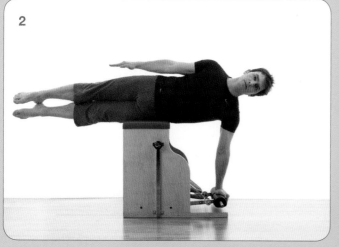

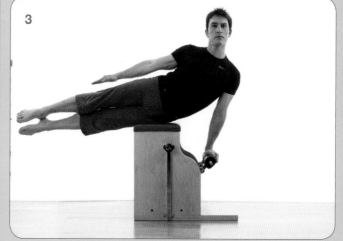

cobra

The Cobra on the Chair is very similar to the Cobra that you have previously learnt on the mat. The resistance of the springs will give you the support required to lift your spine into extension with length, and because of the altered relationship between your arms and your spine you will probably find it a little easier to open up in the front of your hips.

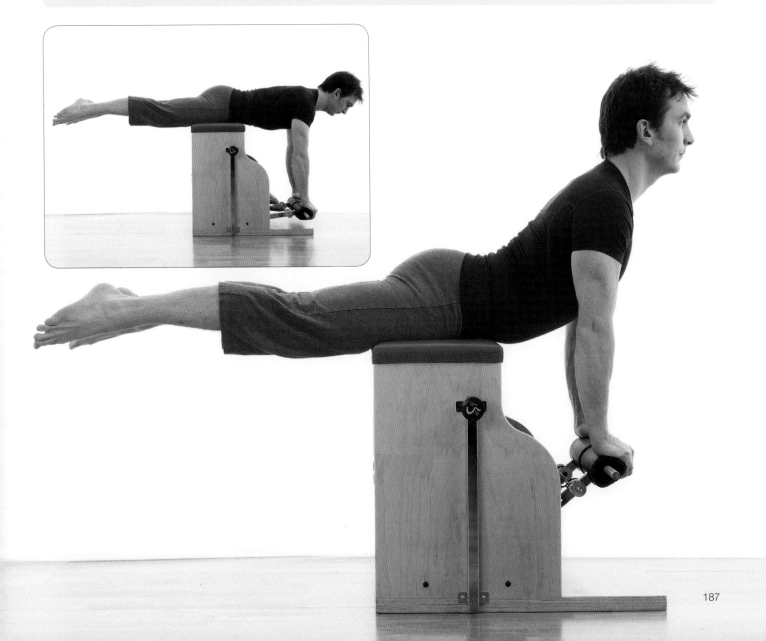

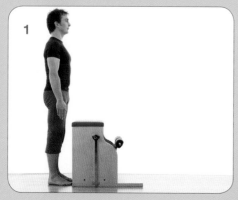

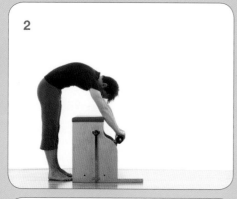

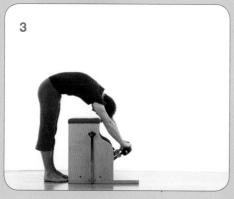

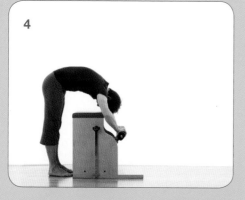

standing roll downs – with arm press

By performing the Beginners' Matwork exercise Roll Downs on the Chair, you will really be able to feel where you are in space, and therefore correct your alignment and positioning. Also, the added resistance of the springs helps to deepen the connection in your core abdominals and will allow you actively to open up and lengthen the muscles of your spine, particularly in the lower back. The added Arm Press also challenges your stability, both in the shoulder girdle area and in your core.

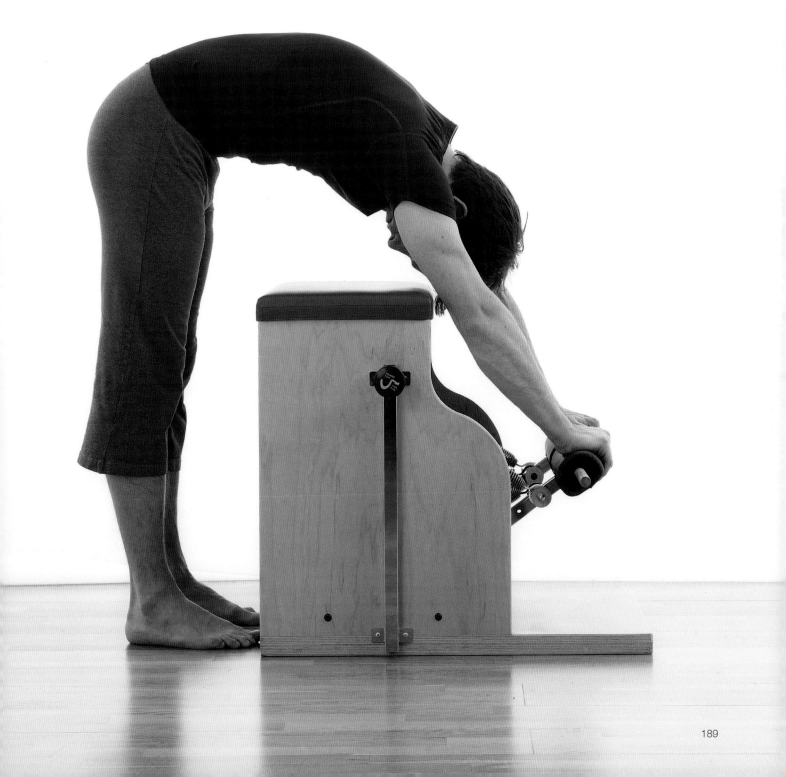

The barrel

The Barrel differs from the pieces of Pilates equipment so far described in that it does not challenge or support the body with spring resistance – there are, in fact, no moving parts at all.

The Barrel can be found in various forms in a Pilates Studio, ranging from the Baby Arc and the Spine Corrector to the much larger Ladder Barrel, which raises the user away from the floor, offering the opportunity for some extremely challenging and impressive exercises. They all follow the same principle of providing a rounded support for certain areas of the spine, whether to challenge balance and improve core control or to help to articulate and mobilise the spine.

We have chosen to demonstrate a variety of exercises using the more challenging Ladder Barrel.

short box series

The following series of exercises enables you to articulate the spine and hips in various planes: a tough challenge for core control and abdominal strength.

Round back

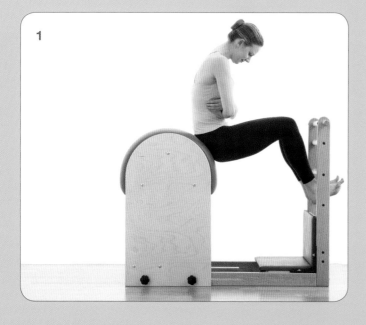

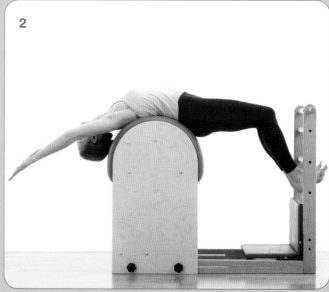

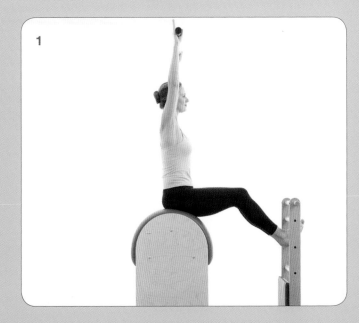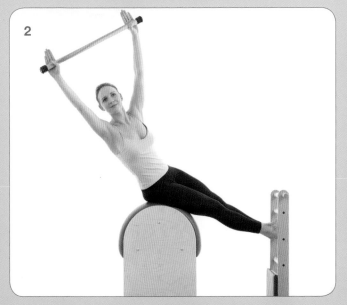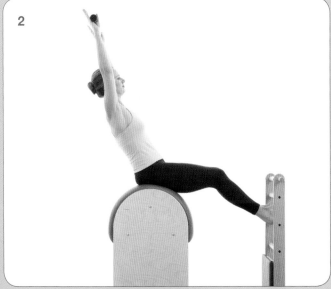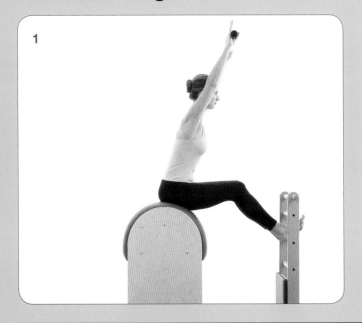

Flat back hinge

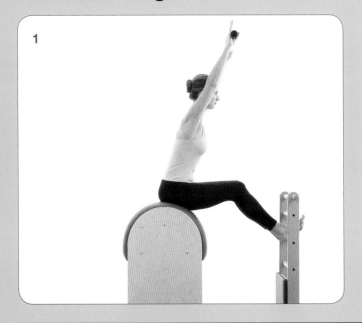

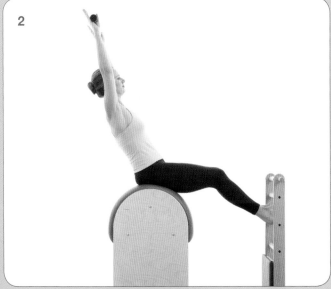

Twist and lean

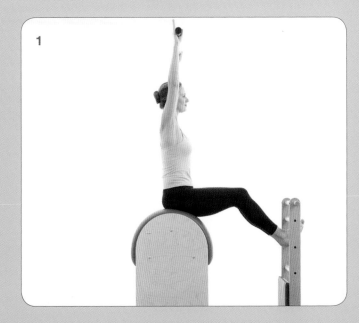

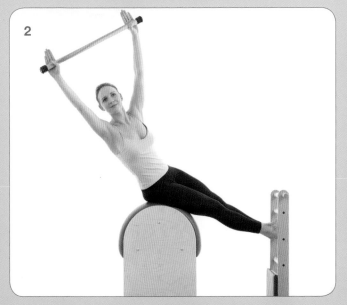

side reach

Far from being an indulgent side stretch, this exercise will challenge your core support and overall spine strength.

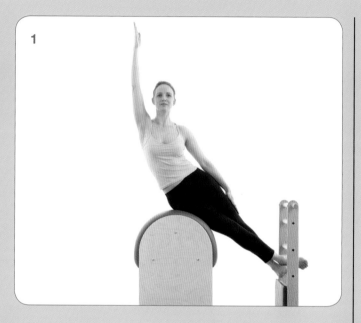

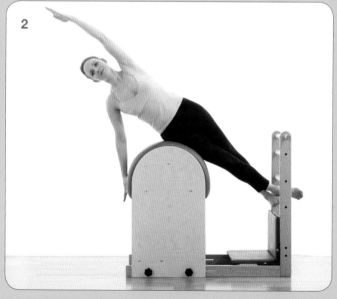

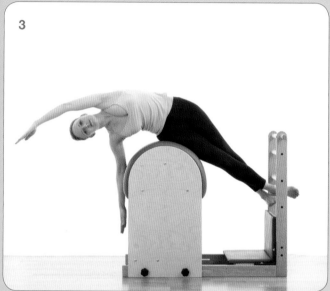

swan dive

Swan Dive on the Ladder Barrel is a great place to perform this back extension exercise. Because of the nature and shape of the Barrel you will find that you are able to take your entire body, hips and spine through from a fully flexed position into a fully extended position.

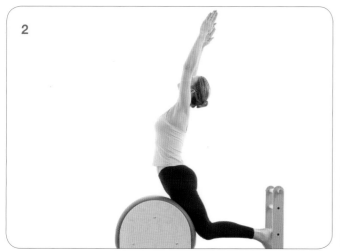

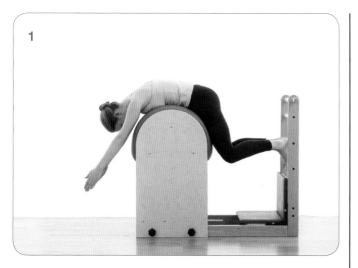

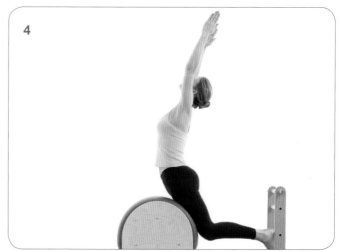

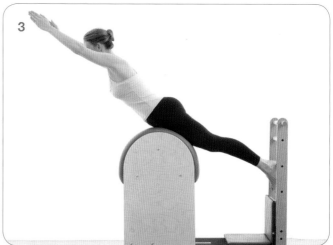

small equipment

Many pieces of portable equipment can be used to enhance and develop the matwork exercises, adding both variety and challenge. These aids offer simplicity coupled with affordability.

The more popular small equipment includes the Band, the Small Ball, the Big Ball, the Toning Circle, the Foam Roller and Free (hand-held) Weights. A selection of exercises for each piece follows to show their individual versatility.

The band

Resistance bands, or stretch bands, are a very popular accessory, commonly used in an array of fitness activities and rehabilitation environments. They can be used to enhance many existing matwork exercises as well as for completely new ones. Many of the exercises using bands offer similar benefits to the resistance studio equipment. There are three distinct ways in which resistance can be employed within exercises:

1. To make difficult exercises easier by providing support and feedback to the parts of the body connected to the band;
2. To change the muscles working within an exercise by changing the direction of forces being applied to the body throughout the exercise;
3. To increase the physical challenge of an exercise further by adding to the resistance already felt from gravity.

The following exercises take advantage of the variety of uses for the band. Many of these exercises may seem similar to some of those in the Beginners' and Intermediate Programmes, but be ready for them to feel quite different!

Bands come in a variety of resistances and lengths. We recommend light to medium resistance bands of around 1.3–2m for use in Pilates exercises.

standing leg press

■ beginners

Improves the muscular recruitment patterns around the hip and the knee joints, while challenging pelvic stability and control.

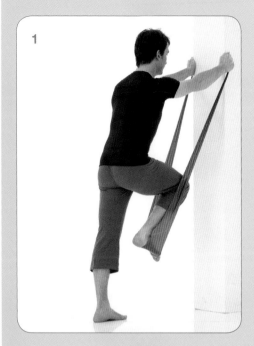

starting position

Stand correctly facing a wall, just over one arm's distance away. Bend your right leg and put your foot on the middle of the band, then press back to the floor. Your feet are in parallel and hip-width apart. Hold either end of the band, reach your arms forwards and place your hands onto the wall at head height. Your whole body should now be leaning forwards on a diagonal line; your head, spine and pelvis remain in neutral alignment.

Maintain an appropriate level of connection to your centre throughout.

action

● Breathe in as you lift the right leg, bending evenly at the hip and knee, aiming the knee up and forwards towards the wall and the heel towards your buttocks.

● Breathe out as you press the foot back down to the floor, again working evenly between the hip and knee.

Repeat up to ten times and then repeat on the other leg.

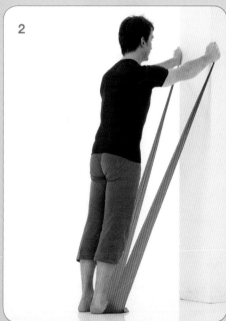

WATCH POINTS

★ Keep your weight balanced evenly through the entire surface area of your supporting foot.

★ Fully lengthen your supporting leg but avoid locking the knee.

★ Maintain the parallel alignment of both legs; ensure that your knees remain facing forwards.

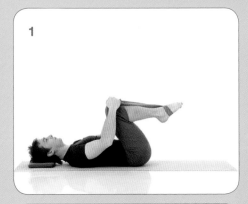

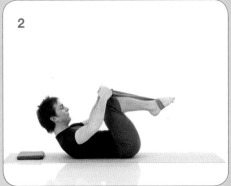

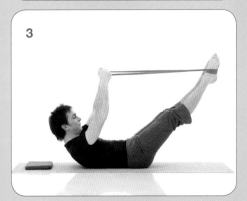

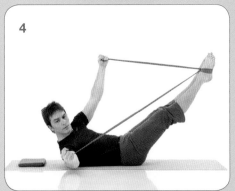

oblique twist

■ intermediate

Challenges the abdominals and upper arms while helping to increase mobility in the spine.

starting position

Align yourself correctly in the Relaxation Position. Double Knee Fold one leg at a time with stability and, keeping your heels connected and your feet softly pointed, open your knees slightly. Wrap the band around both feet and cross it over, taking hold of each end.

Breathe in, preparing your body to move, and, as you breathe out, nod your head and sequentially wheel your neck and upper body off the mat into a Curl Up position. Lengthen your arms forwards and place your hands (holding the band) onto the outside of your knees.

Remain curled up and straighten both legs, pressing your feet into the band on a low diagonal. Connect your inner thighs in the Pilates Stance position. Simultaneously reach your straight arms up and out in front of your shoulders. The band will stretch away in both directions.

Maintain an appropriate level of connection to your centre throughout.

WATCH POINTS

★ Ensure that your pelvis remains grounded in neutral and square throughout; curl up only as far as this can be maintained.

★ Keep both sides of the waist equally long. Avoid 'hitching' your pelvis up towards your ribcage.

★ The rotational movement should come from your head, neck, ribcage and upper back, not the pelvis and hips.

★ Encourage the width across your chest by actively reaching both arms away from your centre line as you rotate.

action

• Breathe in, maintaining the curled-up position, rotate your head and torso to the right and simultaneously open your right arm to the right, stretching the band out wider towards the floor.

• Breathe out and, maintaining the curled-up position, return your head and spine back to the centre and lengthen, releasing your right arm back to the Starting Position.

Repeat up to five times on each side.

To finish, bend the legs back in towards your torso, maintaining the connection of the heels as the knees open. Simultaneously circle the arms out to the side and around, returning to the knees in the Starting Position. Before rolling your upper spine and head back down to the mat, remove the band from your feet and then, maintaining a stable pelvis, return your feet to the mat to finish in the Relaxation Position.

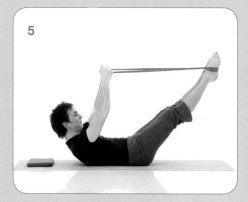

5

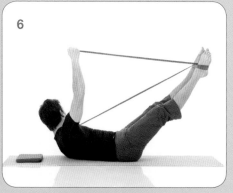

6

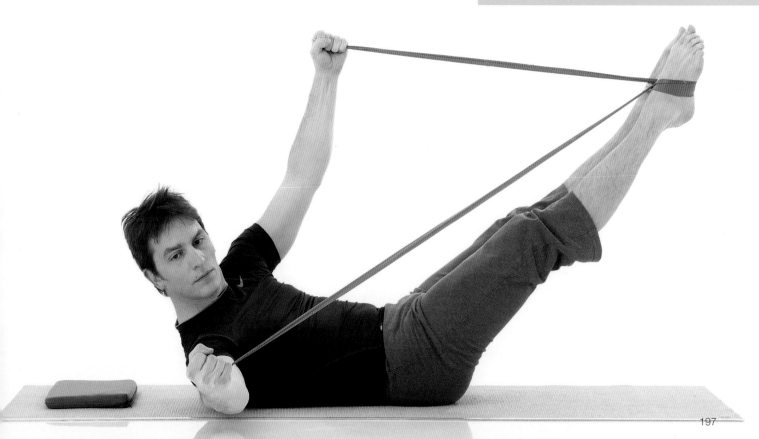

waist twist

intermediate

Promotes good spinal alignment; the band helps to connect the spinal movement to the arm movement, encouraging the shoulders to move freely.

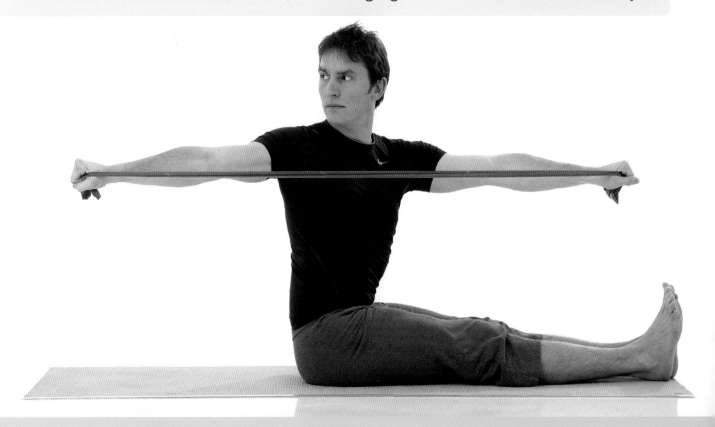

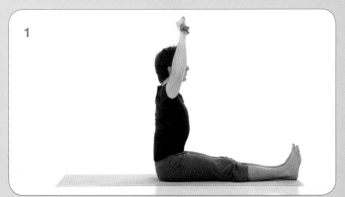

1

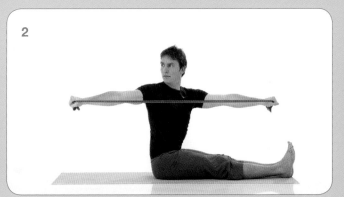

2

starting position

Sit upright with your legs lengthened out in front of your body, your pelvis and spine are in neutral; your legs are parallel with the inner thighs connected and your feet are flexed.

Holding the band in your hands, raise your arms overhead, slightly wider than shoulder-width apart.

If you find it difficult to sit with a neutral pelvis and spine in this position, sit on a cushion or rolled-up towel to help attain the correct alignment.

Maintain an appropriate level of connection to your centre throughout.

action

● Breathe in, preparing your body to move, and lengthen your spine.

● Breathe out as you initiate movement with a turn of the head and rotate your torso fully to the right. Simultaneously, draw the arms apart and down to shoulder height.

● Continue to breathe out fully as you pulse into your position two times, trying to deepen the position each time. Expel all of your breath on the last pulse.

● Breathe in as you return your spine back to the centre and raise your arms once again overhead. Maintain a strong centre and lengthened spine as you do so.

Repeat to the other side and then repeat the whole sequence up to five times.

WATCH POINTS

★ Your pelvis should remain still. Keep the weight even on both sitting bones and maintain their contact to the mat throughout.

★ Focus on connecting to your deep abdominals to help support your spine as you rotate and return.

★ The movement is pure rotation. Continue to keep the spine lengthening vertically and avoid arching in your back or shortening in your waist.

★ Carry your arms with the spine; do not allow them to lead the movement.

★ Encourage width across the chest by actively reaching both arms away from your centre line as your press the arms down.

★ Allow maximum rotation of the head and neck, but ensure length throughout.

★ Keep your feet flexed and fully lengthen both legs but avoid locking your knees.

★ Breathe fully. By the third pulse you should really feel that you are emptying your lungs. As you inhale, fill the lungs up and lengthen the spine to return to the centre.

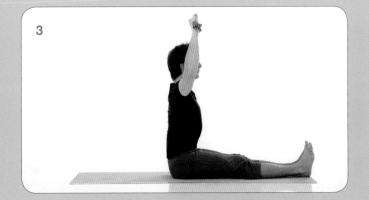

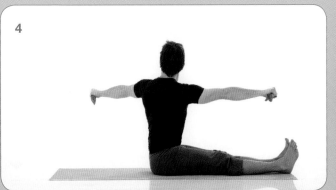

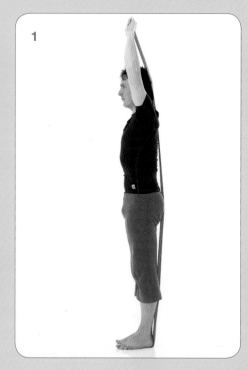

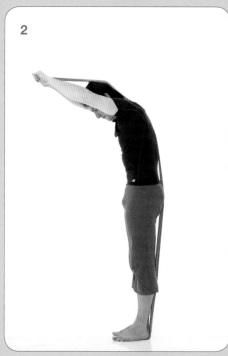

roll downs

beginners

This exercise mobilises the spine and hips. The support and feedback provided by the band make the exercise easier to control.

starting position

Stand tall on the floor (not on your mat) and lengthen your spine into neutral.
Connect your inner thighs in Pilates Stance.
Secure one end of the band underneath your heels and hold the other end with both hands. Reach your arms overhead towards the ceiling.
Keep the band flat and in contact with the back of your pelvis, your upper back and the back of your head.
Maintain an appropriate level of connection to your centre throughout.

action

● Breathe in as you lengthen the back of your neck and nod your head forwards.
● Breathe out as you continue to roll your entire spine forwards and down.
Really make sure that you roll sequentially through each section of your spine and maintain a strong centre. Roll until you can go no further without your hips hinging. Maintain the same relationship between the head and arms throughout, keeping the back of your head and your curved spine and pelvis pressed into the surface of the band.
● Breathe in as you initiate movement with the pelvis, open the front of the hips and begin to wheel your entire spine sequentially back to its upright position; your arms and head should return towards the ceiling at the same time as one another. Repeat up to ten times.

WATCH POINTS

★ Ensure that you roll smoothly and sequentially through each segment of your spine.

★ Maintain length throughout your spine; avoid any shortening or compression of the spine, particularly as you roll down. Remember to connect your deep abdominals to support your spine, and use the band for feedback and support throughout the body.

★ As you roll down, begin the movement with a nod of your head, and as you roll up, begin the movement from your pelvis rolling underneath.

★ Roll directly through your centre line, avoiding any deviations.

★ Maintain an active connection of your inner thighs throughout.

★ It is important to maintain even weight through the feet, paying particular attention not to lift up your heels or you will lose the band!

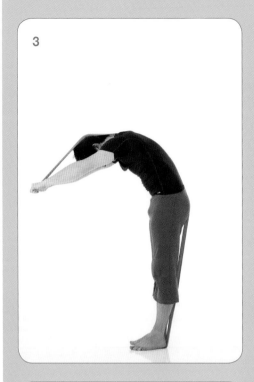

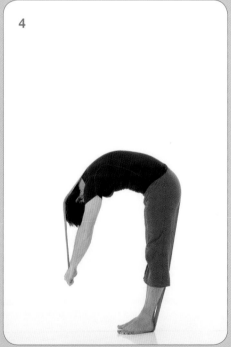

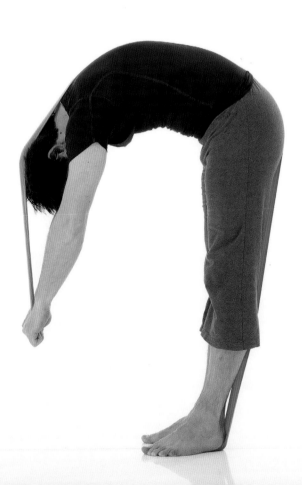

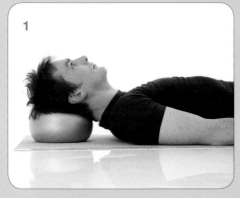

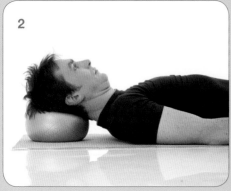

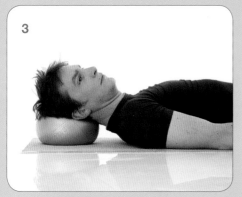

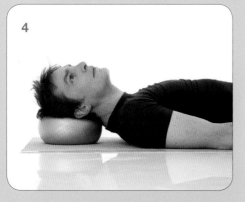

The small ball

In recent years, the Small Ball has become one of the most popular Pilates accessories. There are many different types of ball available in various sizes. We recommend using one between 17.5 and 25cm in diameter, inflated to between 75–80 per cent of its full volume. The smaller balls are generally known as 'Overballs' and a favourite amongst the larger balls is the Triadball(TM).

The benefits of the Small Ball include:

● facilitating a stronger connection to your centre, by helping you focus on more effective recruitment of the key areas involved in the stability process. This often makes the exercise feel deeper and more physically challenging, which actually makes it easier to perform with control;

● assisting in maintaining correct alignment by offering a physical point of reference from which to move;

● challenging joint mobility and control as well as supporting the body and making otherwise difficult exercises easier to perform;

● developing (through its unstable nature and limited base of support) the deep stabilising muscles by challenging the body's balance and control.

This selection of exercises makes full use of the possibilities offered by the Small Ball. Many of them provide useful progressions from or alternatives to exercises in the Beginners' and Intermediate Programmes.

nose circles

█ beginners

Help release tension around the head and neck area, improving your posture.

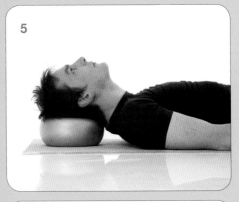

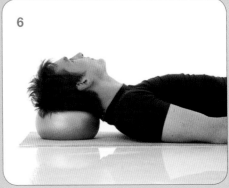

starting position

Please note: the Ball needs to be less inflated for this exercise (50–60 per cent). Align yourself correctly in the Relaxation Position. Raise your head from the mat enough to place the Small Ball underneath. Release your head squarely into the top surface of the Ball. The extra height of the head means there will be an increase in the curvature of your neck. Be sure that you're comfortable and released around your neck and shoulders before moving on.
Maintain an appropriate level of connection to your centre throughout.

action

Breathe naturally throughout.
● Keeping your neck lengthened and released, begin to roll your head on the Ball in small circular motions, first clockwise and then anti-clockwise. Decrease the size of the circle each time and really try to feel your head moving independently from your neck.
Repeat up to ten times in each direction.

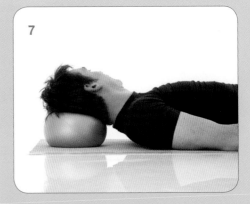

WATCH POINTS

★ Perform the circles slowly and with control but feel released and relaxed as you do so.

★ Try shutting your eyes to help you relax and focus on the movement from the head on top of the spine.

curl ups with arm circles

██ intermediate

Mobilise the upper back, neck and shoulders while strengthening the abdominals through a greater range of movement than in the regular version.

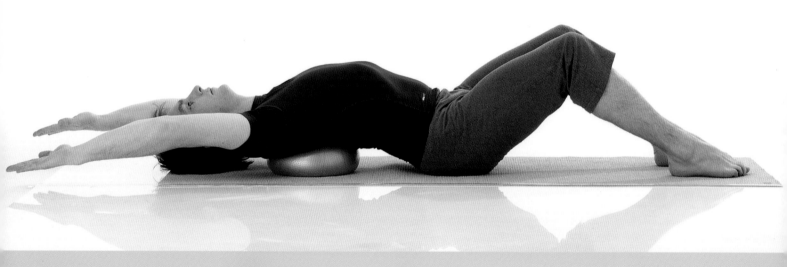

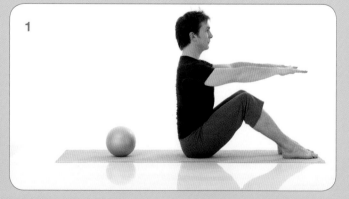

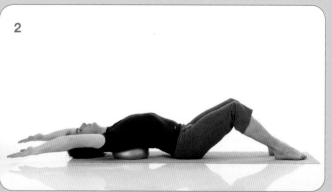

starting position

Sit upright with your knees bent and the soles of your feet grounded on the mat. Your legs are hip-width apart and your pelvis and spine are in neutral. Reach your arms out in front of you, slightly lower than shoulder height and shoulder-width apart. Your arms are lengthened, and your palms are facing down. Place the Ball approximately two hands' distance behind your pelvis. Breathe in, preparing your body to move, and, as you breathe out, sequentially roll your pelvis and spine back onto the Ball so that the middle of the Ball supports your upper back between your shoulder blades. Allow your upper back, neck and head to lengthen into slight extension over the Ball while maintaining a neutral alignment between the lower back and the pelvis. Take care not to let your head hang from the neck; use a small cushion to support the head if necessary. Raise your arms overhead towards the mat, palms facing upwards.

Maintain an appropriate level of connection to your centre throughout.

action

● Breathe out as you circle your arms out to the side and down towards the body, turning your palms down to the mat. Simultaneously lengthen the back of your neck, nod your head forwards and sequentially curl up the upper body; maintain contact of your upper back onto the Ball.

● Breathe in as you sequentially roll your upper spine and head back down over the Ball and raise your arms overhead. Repeat up to ten times.

WATCH POINTS

★ Ensure that your pelvis remains grounded in neutral throughout; curl forwards and arch backwards only as far as this can be maintained.

★ Focus on wheeling your spine away from the Ball vertebra by vertebra.

★ Control the sequential return of your spine back down over the Ball.

★ Allow your collarbones and shoulder blades to widen, but keep a connection of the shoulder blades to the back of the ribcage.

★ Keep the neck long and free from tension. Avoid over-arching the neck and never allow your head to hang or collapse.

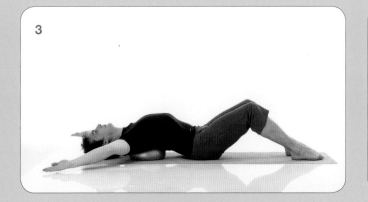

3

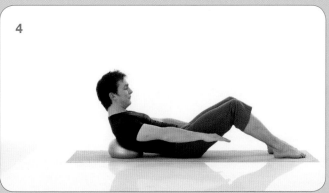

4

the hundred – preparation

■ beginners

Targets the inner thigh muscles, which will be felt more easily using the Small Ball, while continuing to focus on the abdominal connection.

starting position

Align yourself correctly in the Relaxation Position. Double Knee Fold one leg at a time with stability and, keeping your heels connected and your feet softly pointed, open your knees slightly. Position the Ball comfortably in between your knees and gently squeeze your inner thighs.

Breathe in, preparing your body to move, and, as you breathe out, nod your head and sequentially wheel your neck and upper body off the mat into a Curl Up position. Maintaining length in the arms, raise them slightly from the mat.

Maintain an appropriate level of connection to your centre throughout.

action

● Breathe in for a count of five and, remaining curled up, beat the arms up and down five times.
● Breathe out for a count of five, focusing on a full exhalation, and again beat the arms up and down five times.
Repeat up to ten times.
To finish, roll back down to the mat, remove the Ball and then, maintaining a stable pelvis, return your feet to the mat.

WATCH POINTS

★ Ensure that your pelvis remains grounded in neutral throughout.

★ Focus on the ribs gently expanding on the inhalation and drawing together on the exhalation.

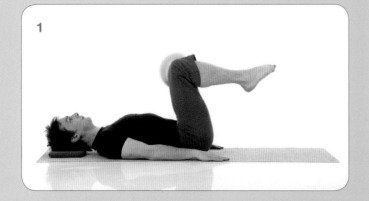

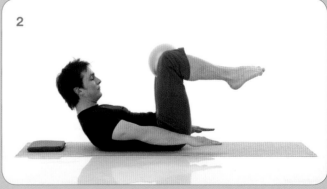

the hundred

intermediate

Follow the instructions for The Hundred – Preparation (opposite).
This time, however, place the Ball in between your ankles and
straighten your legs. Continue to squeeze your inner thighs
together gently, maintaining the placement throughout.

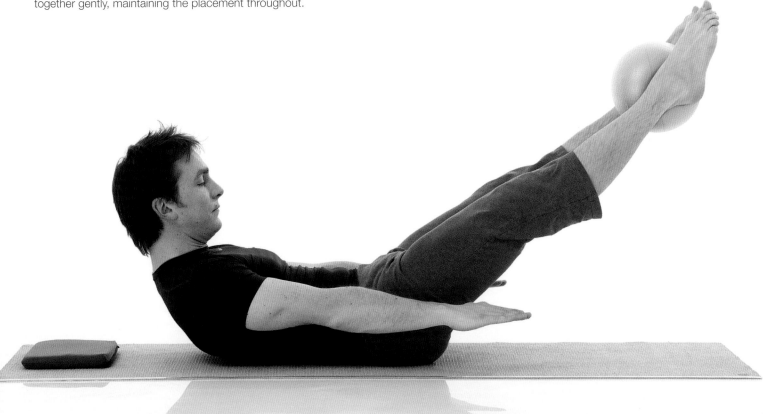

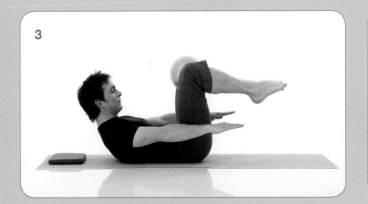

3

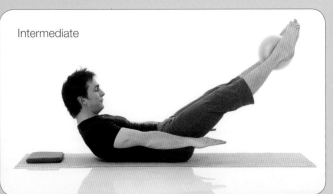

Intermediate

The toning circle

The Toning Circle is a traditional piece of Pilates equipment, often called the Magic Circle. It was originally made in steel, but modern versions are lighter, being made of plastic. Like the Small Ball it can help facilitate a stronger connection to your centre. As well as squeezing the Circle lightly with the inside of the legs, you can also put it around the legs and apply outward pressure to give different connections within the exercise. The size of the Circle means that it can be used with the arms either squeezing together or pulling apart to help change the connection in and around the upper body throughout an exercise.

The following exercises make full use of this versatility, providing useful progressions from or alternatives to exercises covered in the Beginners' and Intermediate Programmes.

arm openings

beginners

Challenge the stability of your pelvis whilst strengthening your inner thighs and mobilise the head, neck and spine.

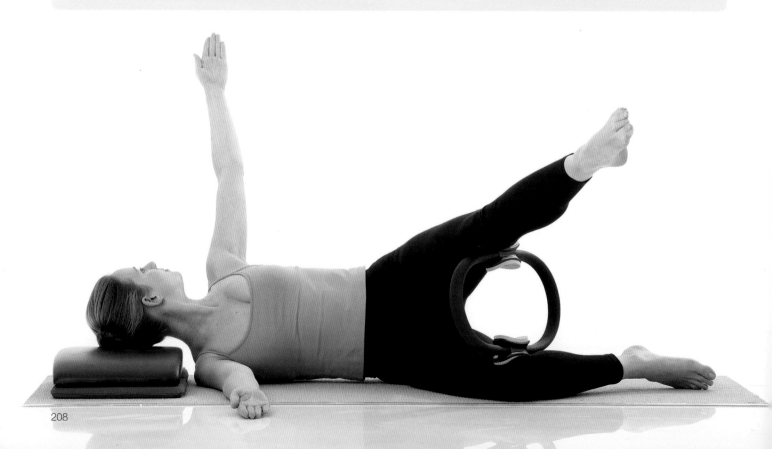

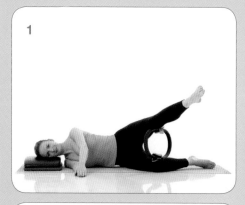

starting position

Lie on your right side and correctly align your pelvis and spine in neutral.
Place a substantial cushion underneath the head to ensure that your head and
neck are in line with your spine. Lengthen both arms out in front of your body at
shoulder height. Your right arm is resting on the mat and your left arm is placed on
top of the right.

Bend both knees in front of you so that your hips and knees are bent to a right
angle. Lift your top leg enough to place the Circle in between your knees, gently
squeezing your inner thighs to maintain this placement, then straighten the top
knee and lengthen your leg away.

Maintain an appropriate level of connection to your centre throughout.

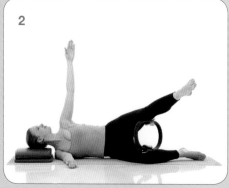

action

● Breathe in as you raise the top arm, keeping it straight and lifting it above the
shoulder joint towards the ceiling; simultaneously roll your head and neck to
face the ceiling.

● Breathe out as you continue to rotate your head, neck and upper spine to the
left; carry your left arm with your spine and open it further towards the mat.
Your knees and pelvis remain still.

● Breathe in as you rotate your spine back to the right, initiating the movement
from your centre. Simultaneously reach your left arm once again above the
shoulder joint and towards the ceiling.

● Breathe out as you rotate and return your spine and arm back to the
Starting Position.

Repeat up to five times, and then repeat on the other side.

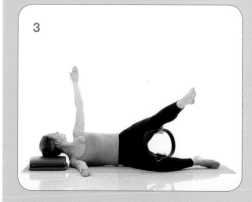

WATCH POINTS

★ Ensure correct alignment in your Side-lying Starting Position: shoulder
above shoulder, hip above hip, knee above knee and foot above foot.

★ Ensure that your pelvis remains stable throughout.

★ Keep only a gentle squeeze on the circle in between your knees; too
much or too little will result in the displacement of the Circle.

★ The movement is ideally pure rotation. Continue to lengthen the
spine; avoid arching in your back or shortening in your waist.

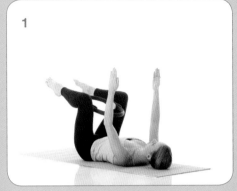

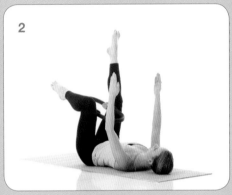

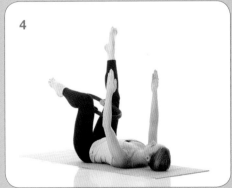

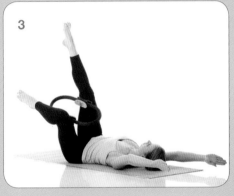

hip rolls plus leg extension and arm reach

intermediate

A challenging coordination exercise that helps encourage spinal rotation while strengthening the abdominals, hips and thighs.

starting position

Align yourself correctly in the Relaxation Position. Double Knee Fold one leg at a time with stability, keeping your legs in parallel and your knees and feet hip-width apart. Raise both arms vertically above your chest, shoulder-width apart, with your palms facing one another.

Place the Circle in between your knees and, keeping your feet the same width apart as your knees, gently squeeze your inner thighs to maintain this placement. Maintain an appropriate level of connection to your centre throughout, along with a light connection to the Circle with the inner thighs.

WATCH POINTS

★ Throughout, focus on the connection of the inner thighs to the Circle as well as maintaining the length through the straightened leg in opposition to the arm reach.

★ Roll your pelvis and your legs directly to the side and avoid any deviation; there should be no shortening on either side of the waist.

action

● Breathe in; keeping your thighs still, straighten your right leg and softly point your foot towards the ceiling.

● Breathe out as you begin to rotate your pelvis and legs to the left from a strong centre. Maintain length through your extended right leg as the right side of the pelvis lifts slightly off the mat. Simultaneously, lengthen and reach your arms overhead towards the floor, softening your breastbone and closing your ribs as you do so.

● Breathe in and return your pelvis, legs and arms back to the centre, initiating the movement from a strong centre.

Repeat to the other side and then repeat the whole sequence up to five times.

To finish, remove the Circle and, maintaining a stable pelvis, return your feet to the mat to end in the Relaxation Position.

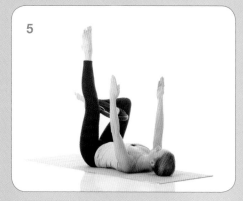

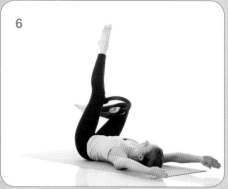

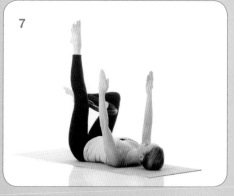

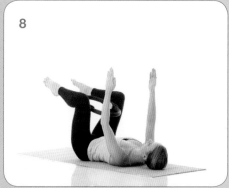

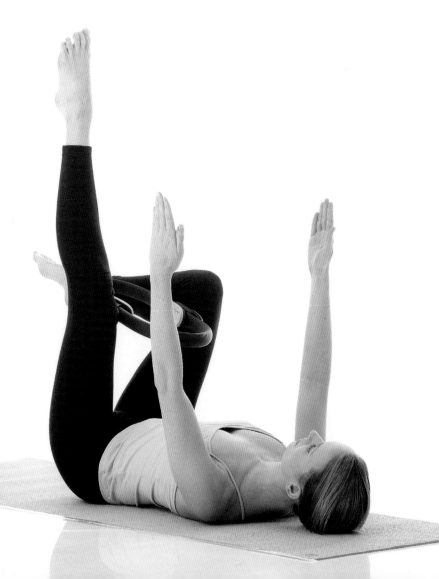

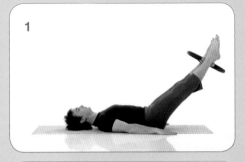

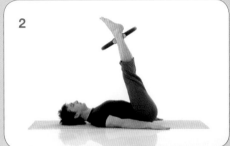

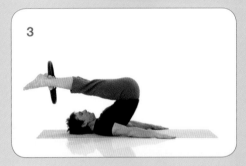

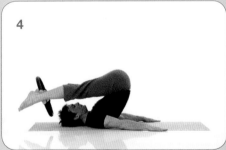

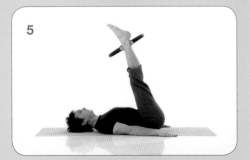

roll over with leg squeeze and pull

■ intermediate

Promotes mobilisation of the hips and spine and helps develop strength along the front of the body and legs and the back of your arms.

starting position

Align yourself correctly in the Relaxation Position. Double Knee Fold one leg at a time with stability, position the Circle comfortably in between your ankles and softly point your feet.

Keeping your legs in parallel, straighten them directly above your pelvis and then lower them to a point where you can still maintain a neutral pelvis and spine; do not allow your lower back to arch.

Maintain a connection of your inner thighs and a gentle and consistent squeeze of the Circle throughout the entire exercise.

Maintain an appropriate level of connection to your centre throughout.

WATCH POINTS

★ Continue to press your legs towards one another, maintaining consistent but gentle pressure into the Circle throughout. Make sure that you do not grip in your hip area or lock your knees. It is important not to squeeze too hard.

★ Initiate the movement from a strong centre and maintain this connection throughout.

★ Focus on maintaining length in the spine, avoiding any compression, especially as the legs lower in the Roll Over position.

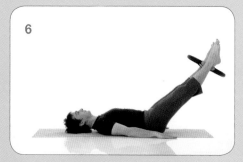

action

- Breathe in as you lengthen your legs and begin to draw your legs in towards your body, keeping your pelvis down for as long as possible.
- Breathe out as you allow your pelvis and spine to roll sequentially off the mat, drawing the legs up and over your torso until they are parallel with the mat. Make sure that you do not roll too far; there should not be any pressure on the neck and head or tension in the shoulders.
- Breathe in and, without deepening the curve of the spine, attempt to lower both legs a little nearer the mat.
- Breathe out and sequentially roll the spine and pelvis back down along the mat. Keep the legs close to the front of the body until your pelvis and spine have returned to neutral.
- Still breathing out, lower the legs away from your torso, towards the mat as far as possible without losing your neutral spinal alignment.

Repeat up to five times.

To finish, return the legs directly above the pelvis and then bend the knees. Remove the Circle and, maintaining a stable pelvis, return your legs one at a time to the mat to end in the Relaxation Position.

Variation: Leg Pull

Repeat the above exercise, this time placing your ankles inside the Circle and maintaining constant pressure outwards as you perform the exercise.

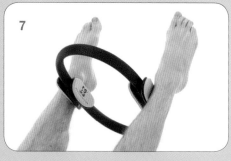

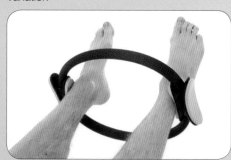

Variation

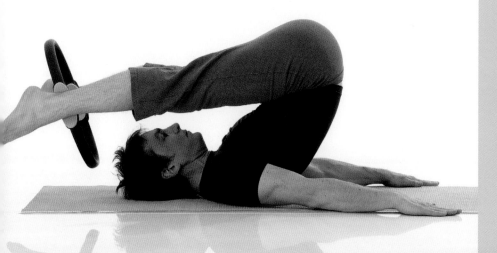

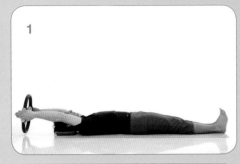

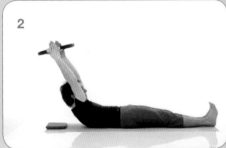

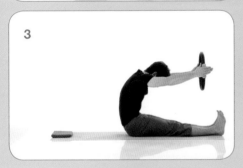

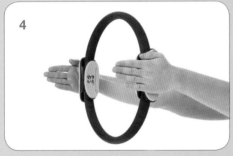

roll up with arm press

intermediate

The arm press against the Circle helps free tension around the neck and shoulders.

starting position

Lie on your back with both legs straight and connected together in parallel with your feet flexed. Your pelvis and spine are in neutral. Hold the Circle in between your lengthened hands and, gently squeezing it, raise your arms overhead, maintaining openness across the chest. Continue this connection of the arms to the Circle and keep the pressure consistently steady throughout the entire exercise. Maintain an appropriate level of connection to your centre throughout.

action

● Breathe in as you raise your arms and simultaneously begin to roll up from your head, neck and upper back.

● Breathe out as you continue to roll the rest of the spine, sequentially wheeling it off the mat, one vertebra at a time. Lengthen the C-Curved spine over your legs. Reach the arms forward, ensuring that they maintain their relationship with your neck and head.

● Breathe in as you begin to roll the pelvis and spine back along the mat, ensuring that you initiate the movement from the pelvis.

● Breathe out as you continue to wheel the whole spine sequentially down onto the mat, returning the head and the arms on the final part of your exhalation. Repeat up to ten times.

WATCH POINTS

★ Focus on the control of the movement with your breath.

★ Keep the whole movement even-paced and flowing.

The big ball

The Big Ball is extremely popular in a variety of fitness-training environments. Most commonly known as Swiss Ball or Physio Ball, it is a great way of adding challenge and fun to your Pilates sessions.

When purchasing a Big Ball, there are two main factors to consider:

1. The Ball should be made from 'anti-burst' material. Many of the exercises you can do on the Big Ball involve supporting the majority of your body weight on the Ball from elevated positions, such as sitting. It therefore needs to be designed to support more than your own weight – we suggest at least double. The material must also resist tearing so that any puncture that could occur when the Ball is under pressure does not result in it bursting like a balloon, potentially resulting in serious injury. Buy the most durable Ball available, inspect its surface regularly and make sure you use it away from any sharp obstacles.

2. The size of the Ball is important for safe and correct use. Most people should use a Ball of between 55 and 65cm in diameter inflated to 85–100 per cent of the maximum recommended volume. Over-inflating a Big Ball is dangerous and, irrespective of any anti-burst capabilities, can lead to the Ball bursting. A rough guide to finding the right diameter is to sit on the Ball with your feet flat on the floor and check that your hips are slightly higher than your knees.

The Benefits of the Big Ball

● Its unstable nature helps develop the deep stabilising muscles by challenging the body's balance and control.
● It can assist in maintaining correct alignment, offering a physical point of reference from which to move.
● Working from its raised surface changes the range of movement in many familiar exercises – increasing the challenge on joint mobility and control or providing greater support for the body, making a harder exercise easier to perform and understand.

The following exercises provide useful progressions from or alternatives to similar exercises you have covered in the Beginners' and Intermediate Programmes.

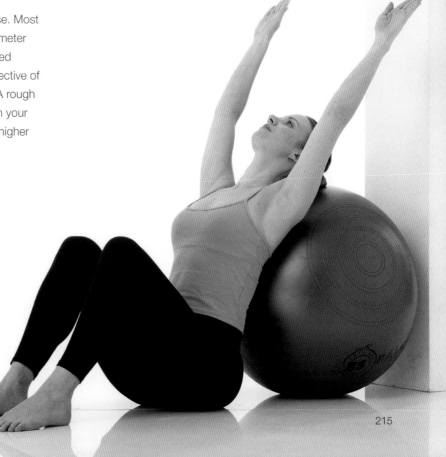

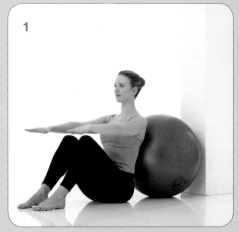

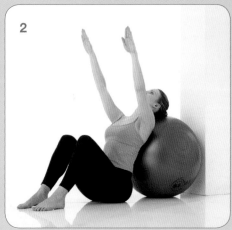

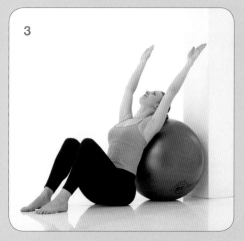

arm circles back over the big ball

■ beginners

Help release tension in the upper back, neck and shoulders, allowing you to mobilise sequentially without putting strain on the abdominal area.

starting position

Sit upright with your knees bent and the soles of your feet grounded on the mat. Your legs are hip-width apart and your pelvis and spine are in neutral. Reach your arms out in front of you, slightly lower than shoulder height and shoulder-width apart. Your arms are lengthened, and your palms are facing down. The Big Ball is placed between your back and a wall.

Breathe in, preparing your body to move, and, as you breathe out, sequentially roll your upper back, neck and head. Allow your upper back, neck and head to lengthen into slight extension over the Ball while maintaining a neutral alignment between the lower back and the pelvis. Take care not to let your head hang from the neck; use a small cushion to support the head if necessary. Raise your arms overhead towards the wall, palms facing upwards.

action

● Breathe out as you circle your arms out to the side and down towards the body, turning your palms down to the mat.

● Breathe in as you raise your arms overhead, returning to the Starting Position. Repeat the action five times and then reverse the movement of the arms for a further five repetitions.

To finish, breathe out as you circle the arms down and simultaneously nod your head and sequentially curl your spine forwards. Restack your spine to return to the Starting Position.

WATCH POINTS

★ Ensure that your pelvis remains grounded in neutral throughout. Arch backwards only as far as this can be maintained.

★ Allow your collarbones and shoulder blades to widen, but keep a connection of the shoulder blades to the back of the ribcage.

★ Keep the neck long and free from tension. Avoid over-arching the neck and never allow your head to hang or collapse.

★ Focus on wheeling your spine away from the Ball vertebra by vertebra.

★ Control the sequential return of your spine back down over the Ball.

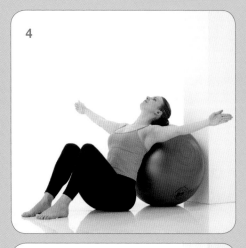

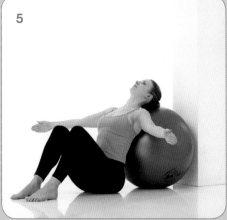

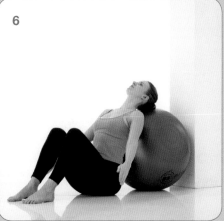

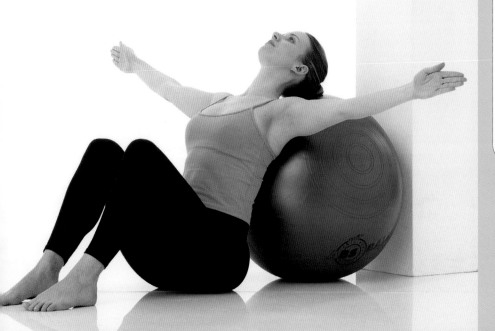

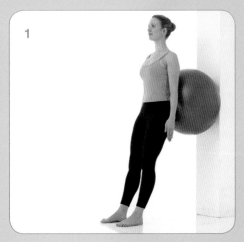

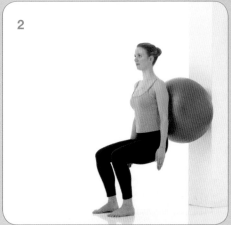

sliding down the wall

■ beginners

Helps strengthen and balance the leg muscles. Mobilises and coordinates the hip, knee and ankle joints while challenging the stability of the spine.

starting position

Stand tall with your back to a wall and place the Big Ball between your lower back and the wall. Place your feet in parallel and hip-width apart; your feet should be slightly forwards of your pelvis, so that when your knees are bent to a right angle, your knees do not go beyond your toes. Although you are leaning into the Ball your spine is lengthened and in neutral. Allow your arms to lengthen down by the sides of your body.

Maintain an appropriate level of connection to your centre throughout.

action

● Breathe in, lengthen your spine and bend your knees; as you lower towards the floor, the Ball will roll smoothly up your spine. Maintain your vertical position and your neutral pelvis and spine as you lower.

● Breathe out and, grounding your feet down into the floor, straighten your legs and return up, lengthening your spine as you do so. Feel the Ball naturally roll back down to where it began in your lower back.

Repeat up to ten times.

WATCH POINTS

★ Maintain a neutral pelvis and spine throughout. Remain long in your waist and keep a sense of your spine lengthening up and away from the floor.

★ Avoid lowering your pelvis below the level of your knees.

★ Maintain correct alignment of your legs; ensure that your ankles and knees remain in line with your hips.

diamond press

■ beginners

Helps develop spinal mobility, particularly in and around the upper back. The Big Ball promotes this by heightening awareness of this area.

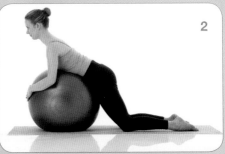

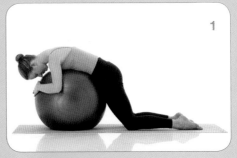

starting position

Kneel upright and place the Ball in front of your body. Lean onto the Ball, resting your thighs against it, and then lengthen and curl your spine forwards over the Ball. Your pelvis, abdominal area, ribcage and chest should all be supported by the Ball. Create a diamond shape with the arms: place the fingertips together, palms down onto the Ball and open your elbows. Rest your forehead on the backs of the hands.

Maintain an appropriate level of connection to your centre throughout.

action

● Breathe in, preparing your body to move.
● Breathe out as you lift first your head, then your neck and then your chest away from the Ball. Feel your lower ribs remaining in contact with the Ball, but open your chest and focus on directing it forwards.
● Breathe in as you hold this lengthened and stable position.
● Breathe out as you return your chest and head forwards and downwards, over the Ball.

Repeat up to ten times.

WATCH POINTS

★ Initiate the back extension by lengthening and lifting your head first, and then your neck. When your head and neck are in line with your spine you can begin to open and lift your chest.

★ Keep your lower ribs in contact with the Ball as you lift up; this will ensure that you don't lift too far and compress your lower spine. The length throughout the spine is far more important than the height of extension that you achieve.

★ Avoid too much pressure down into the arms; they are there to support you lightly and not to press you up.

★ The Ball should remain still throughout.

press ups

intermediate

Strengthen the arms, chest and shoulders, and also help develop strength and stability along the spine and the back of the legs.

starting position

Lie forwards on the Ball; the Ball supports the front of both thighs. Place your hands on the mat directly underneath your shoulders and fully straighten your arms. Your pelvis and spine are correctly aligned in neutral. Lengthen your legs directly behind you, slightly turned out, with the inner thighs connected; softly point your feet. Maintain an appropriate level of connection to your centre throughout.

action

● Breathe in and bend your elbows, directing them out wide in line with the chest. As you remain strong and stable in your centre, your entire body will lower towards the mat. Your legs will reactively rise slightly and the Ball should remain still.
● Breathe out as you straighten your elbows, pressing your body back up to the Starting Position.
Repeat up to five times.

WATCH POINTS

★ Maintain a neutral pelvis and spine throughout. Your spine must also maintain its relationship with your legs. Your spine lowers towards the mat and presses away from it as a result of the action occurring in your elbows and shoulder girdle.

★ It is essential to maintain a good abdominal connection to avoid your pelvis or your ribcage dipping down towards the mat.

★ Maintain a firm connection of the shoulder blades to the back of your ribcage.

★ When bending your elbows, focus on lengthening your body and working your arms away from a strong centre, keeping your chest open.

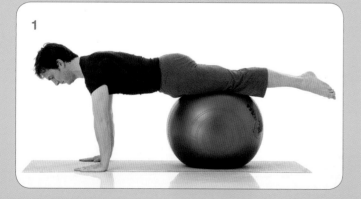

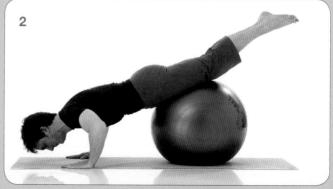

The foam roller

The Foam Roller is a highly effective and versatile piece of equipment that has many applications in the Pilates environment. Various types of Roller are available from different manufacturers, all very similar in construction, although some use a higher-density foam to make them harder-wearing and less likely to lose their shape.

The most important points to consider are size and shape. Foam Rollers usually come in a diameter of 10cm or 15cm. For Pilates exercises we generally recommend the larger 15cm diameter. In terms of length, you basically need the Roller to be longer than your body length, including your neck and head – so, if you are less than 1.75m tall, a standard 90cm-long Roller should suffice. If you are taller you may need a slightly longer Roller in order to support your head, torso and sacrum comfortably when lying on it.

The Benefits of the Foam Roller

● Working from the raised surface of the Roller changes the range of movement in many familiar exercises. This can be used to increase the challenge on joint mobility and control or to provide greater support for the body, making a harder exercise easier to perform and understand.
● Its unstable nature, coupled with the reduced base of support it offers between the body and the floor, is great for challenging the body's ability to maintain balance and control, which is highly effective in developing functional use of the deep stabilising muscles.
● It helps you maintain correct alignment by offering a moving reference point or guide throughout the movement being performed.

The following exercises make full use of the Foam Roller's various applications. Some provide useful progressions from or alternatives to similar exercises you have covered in the Beginners' and Intermediate Programmes.

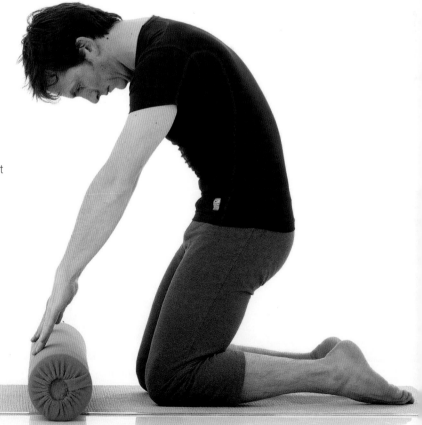

knee folds

■ beginners

> Increase the challenge of maintaining stablilty between the pelvis and spine while promoting independent movement of the leg at the hip joint.

starting position

Align yourself correctly in the Relaxation Position on the Roller. Ensure that your head, ribcage and pelvis are all supported by the Roller and that your feet are placed in parallel and hip-width apart on the floor. Either lengthen your arms alongside the Roller on the mat, or bend your elbows and place your hands lightly on the front of your pelvis.

action

• Breathe in, preparing your body to move.
• Breathe out as you lift your right foot off the mat and fold the knee up towards your body.
• Breathe in, maintain the position and stay centred.
• Breathe out as you slowly return the leg back down and your foot to the mat.
Repeat five times with each leg.

WATCH POINTS

★ Keep your pelvis and spine still and centred throughout; focus on your leg moving in isolation from the rest of your body. Be especially careful as you initially begin to lift your leg.

★ Although the Roller may roll ever so slightly and your body may slightly adjust as a reaction, do try to keep both the Roller and your body still without becoming rigid.

★ Fold your knee in as far as you can without disturbing the pelvis and losing neutral.

★ Keep your chest and the front of your shoulders open and avoid any tension in your neck area.

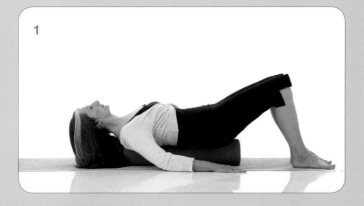

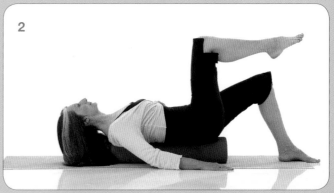

ribcage closure

■ beginners

Builds awareness of spinal stability while promoting mobility and release around your shoulders.

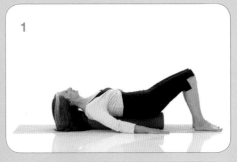

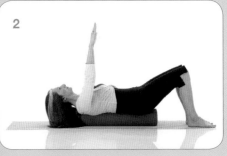

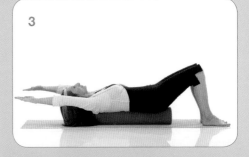

starting position

Align yourself correctly in the Relaxation Position on the Roller. Ensure that your head, ribcage and pelvis are all supported by the Roller and your feet are placed in parallel and hip-width apart on the floor. Lengthen your arms alongside the Roller on the mat; probably only your hands will be in actual contact with the mat. Maintain an appropriate level of connection to your centre throughout.

action

● Breathe in and raise both arms to a vertical position above your chest, palms facing forwards.
● Breathe out. Maintaining a stable and still spine, continue to reach both arms overhead towards the floor. Keep your neck long and encourage the softening and the closing of the ribcage during this exhalation. Your shoulder blades should naturally glide upwards on the back of your ribcage as your arms rise. Although they should not over-elevate, it is important not to block their movement by depressing them down your back. Simply allow them to move naturally and without tension.
● Breathe in as you return the arms above your chest. Feel your ribcage heavy and your chest open.
● Breathe out and lower the arms, returning them to the mat and lengthening them by the sides of your body.
Repeat up to ten times.

WATCH POINTS

★ Keep your pelvis and spine stable and still throughout. Be particularly careful not to allow your upper spine to arch as you reach your arms overhead.

★ During the exhalation encourage stability in your torso and focus on the closing and softening of the ribcage.

★ Fully lengthen your arms, but avoid locking your elbows.

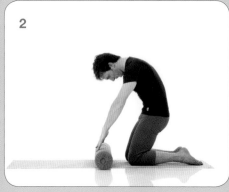

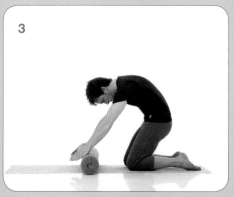

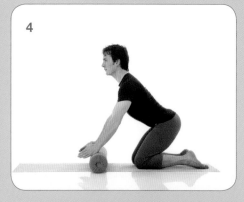

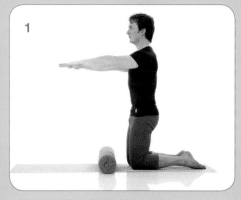

the cat

▨ intermediate

Mobilises the entire spine, the hips and the shoulders and helps develop flowing movement throughout the body using the Roller to guide and facilitate this.

starting position

Kneel upright and place the Roller in front of your knees. Lengthen your pelvis and spine in neutral and raise your arms directly in front of your chest at shoulder height and shoulder-width apart.

Maintain an appropriate level of connection to your centre throughout.

action

● Breathe in, preparing your body to move, and lengthen your spine.
● Breathe out, nod your head and begin sequentially to roll down through your spine while rolling the pelvis under and back, slightly bending your knees to take your buttocks towards your heels. Simultaneously reach your arms down and place your hands on the Roller. As you deepen your C-Curve and direct your buttocks further back, the Roller will roll forwards slightly in opposition.
● Breathe in and keep the Roller still as you begin to roll the pelvis behind you and gently arch your spine all the way from your lower back to your neck. Maintain length and a sense of opposition between the crown of the head and the sitting bones.
● Breathe out as you roll the Roller further away from you by hinging your arched spine down towards the floor from your hips. Ensure that your thigh bones remain still and the arch in your spine remains unchanged. As your arms roll along the Roller allow your palms to turn to face one another.
● Breathe in. First roll your pelvis under and then curl your entire spine back into a C-Curve position. Then unfurl the spine and re-stack back up to your upright position; as you return your spine to vertical, raise your arms back to the Starting Position.

Repeat up to ten times.

WATCH POINTS

★ Focus on connecting to your deep abdominals to help support your spine as it curls and extends sequentially.

★ The Roller will roll forwards as a reaction to your spine, pelvis and hips deepening into a C-Curve, and not simply because your arms are pushing it.

★ Roll directly through the centre line.

★ Keep a relationship between the shoulders and the back of your ribcage. Neither force them to depress, nor allow them to over-elevate, especially when reaching forwards.

★ Beware not to curl forwards excessively from the head and neck; remember you are looking for a balanced curve in the spine. Keep your neck long and free from tension throughout.

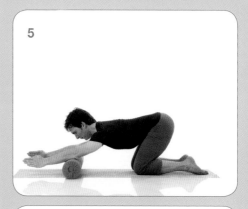

5

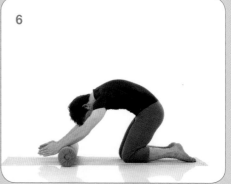

6

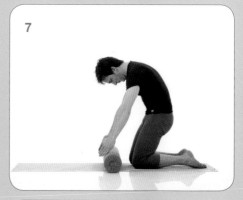

7

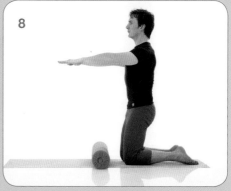

8

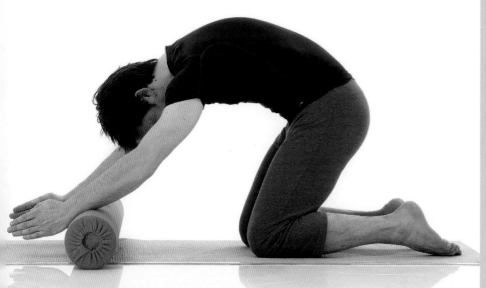

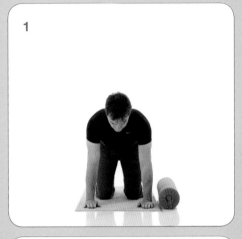

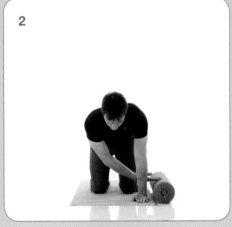

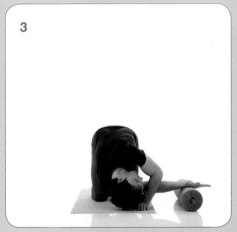

threading the needle

■ intermediate

Mobilises the spine with rotational movement; also helps promote both mobility and stability around the shoulder joints with flowing movement throughout.

starting position

Align yourself correctly in the Four-point Kneeling Position. Place the Roller on the floor next to your left arm, parallel to your lengthened spine.

Maintain an appropriate level of connection to your centre throughout.

action

● Breathe in and lift your right hand off the mat, turning your palm up and reaching it across to your left, behind your left forearm, to place the back of your right hand on top of the Roller. Simultaneously turn your head and torso to the left.

● Breathe out and, bending the elbow of the supporting left arm, allow your torso to increase its rotation, lowering your right shoulder and ear towards the mat. As this happens the Roller will roll away to the left with the right arm.

● Breathe in; return to the Starting Position, maintaining stability and length through the spine as the Roller returns with the body. Remove your right hand from the Roller and continue bringing the arm out to the right side of the body, now rotating the head and torso to the right. Open fully across the front of your chest and shoulders.

Repeat up to five times and then repeat on the other side.

WATCH POINTS

★ Maintain length and support in the spine as it rotates.

★ Avoid curling the spine forwards or arching it back as it rotates. Your body lowers towards the mat and lifts away from it as a result of the bending of your supporting elbow and the hinging in your hip joints.

★ The Roller will roll as a reaction to your spine rotating, and not simply because your arm is pressing it.

★ The contact of the back of your hand onto the Roller is light; do not bear any weight through this hand.

★ The rotation of the spine is sequential; initiate with the head to begin and return by initiating with the centre.

★ Allow the head to rotate accordingly with the rest of the spine.

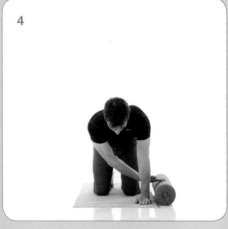

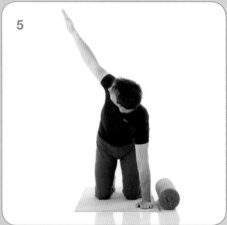

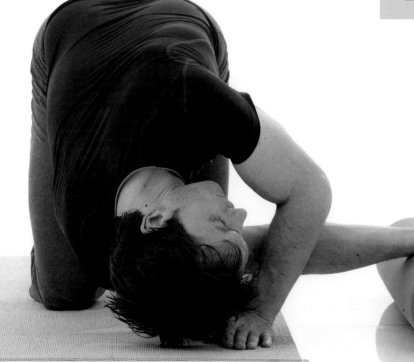

Free weights

Hand-held weights come in various shapes and sizes. The application of Free-weight resistance training is generally used to increase muscular output during the movements being performed. Training techniques vary tremendously, but generally strength training comprises working with heavier weights and a lower number of repetitions, while muscular endurance training generally requires higher repetitions and lighter weights.

The primary reason for working with Free Weights in a Pilates environment is to challenge the integrity of the movement. The added resistance will increase the challenge to joint stability and make it harder to focus on the opposition needed to maintain suitable control of the movement. For this reason, the weights used should be light enough to allow the movement still to be performed correctly. Adding resistance to an exercise is widely believed to improve bone health (see page 248).

Practise the exercises first without weights or holding small balls to refine your technique. When you feel ready, you can try using light weights, gradually building up to heavier weights. How heavy you go to really depends on your individual strength and on the exercise being performed. Essentially, what is important is that the quality of the movement should be challenged, but never compromised!

If you don't have weights available you can hold small (filled) plastic water bottles in each hand, but be mindful of your grip and wrist alignment.

The following Pilates exercises are often performed with hand weights. When considering whether to add weights to other arm movements, ensure that you don't lose sight of the movement intentions of the standard exercise.

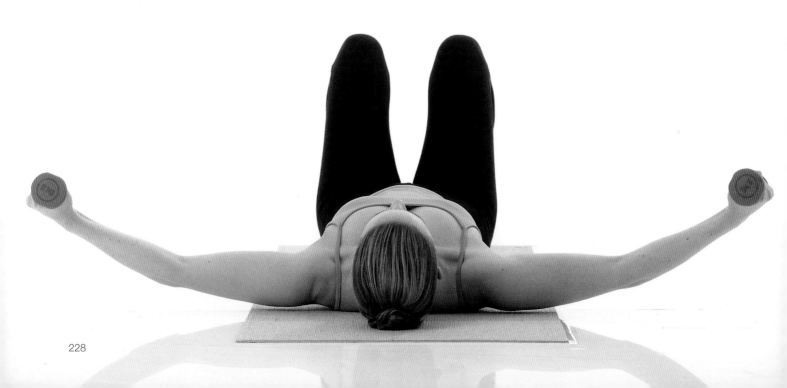

flys

■ beginners

Encourage openness across the chest and shoulders while promoting stability in the upper back, neck and shoulder regions.

Equipment Hand-held weights up to approximately 2kg.

starting position

Align yourself correctly in the Relaxation Position. Holding a weight in each hand, raise both arms vertically above your chest, shoulder-width apart, with your palms facing one another.

Slightly bend your elbows, rounding your arms and opening your chest, and bring the weights into contact with one another, directly over the centre of your chest. Maintain an appropriate level of connection to your centre throughout.

action

● Breathe in and, maintaining the shape of your arms, open them directly out to the sides, lowering the weights close to the mat, but not all of the way.

● Breathe out as you return the arms with control back to the Starting Position. Repeat up to ten times.

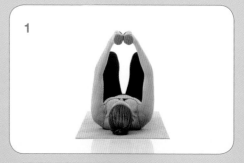

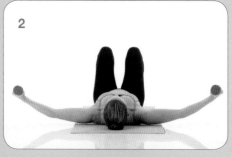

WATCH POINTS

★ Keep your pelvis and spine stable and still throughout. Be particularly careful not to allow your upper spine to arch as you open your arms.

★ As the arms open, ensure that they remain level with the shoulder joints.

★ During the exhalation encourage stability in your torso and focus on the closing and softening of the ribcage.

★ Keep your neck long and free from tension; your head remains still and heavy throughout.

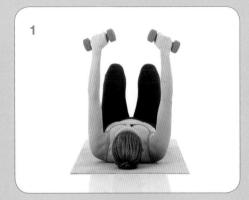

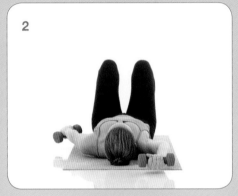

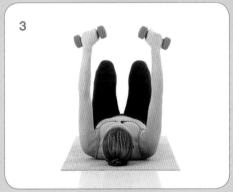

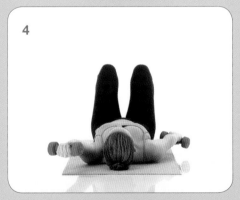

backstroke arms

beginners

Encourages control and release across the chest and shoulders while challenging stability in the upper back, neck and shoulder regions.

Equipment Hand-held weights up to approximately 1.5kg.

starting position

Align yourself correctly in the Relaxation Position. Holding a weight in each hand, lengthen both arms and raise them vertically above your chest, shoulder-width apart, with your palms facing forwards.

Maintain an appropriate level of connection to your centre throughout.

action

- Breathe in, preparing your body to move.
- Breathe out. Maintaining a stable and still spine, reach your right arm overhead towards the floor and lower your left arm down by the side of your body towards the mat. Keep your neck long and encourage the softening and the closing of the ribcage during this exhalation.
- Breathe in as you return both arms to vertical, above your chest. Feel your ribcage heavy and your chest open.

Repeat on the other side and then repeat the whole sequence up to five times.

WATCH POINTS

★ Keep your pelvis and spine stable and still throughout. Be particularly careful not to allow your upper spine to arch as you reach your arm overhead.

★ During the exhalation encourage stability in your torso and focus on the closing and softening of the ribcage.

bicep press

■ beginners

Helps strengthen the arms and shoulders while challenging spinal stability and control.

Equipment Hand-held weights up to approximately 3.5kg.

starting position

Stand tall on the floor (not on your mat) and lengthen your spine into neutral. Your legs are either parallel and hip-width apart, or connected in Pilates Stance. Hold a weight in each hand and lengthen your arms down by the sides of your body with your palms facing in towards you.
Maintain an appropriate level of connection to your centre throughout.

action

● Breathe in and, keeping your upper arms still, bend your elbows and draw your hands up towards the shoulders, turning the palms in to face your body.
● Breathe out as you straighten both elbows and raise your arms upwards overhead, turning your palms to face one another as you do so.
● Breathe in as you bend your elbows, lowering the arms and once again drawing the hands down towards the fronts of the shoulders.
● Breathe out and, once again keeping your upper arms still, straighten and lower your arms, turning your palms into the Starting Position. Repeat up to ten times.

WATCH POINTS

★ Continue to maintain a stable and lengthened, vertical position of your pelvis and spine throughout.

★ Maintain correct wrist alignment: keep your hands and wrists in line with your forearm and avoid rolling your fists away or in towards you.

★ Fully straighten your arms but avoid locking the elbows.

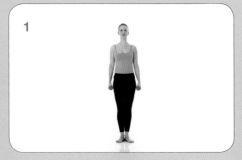

1
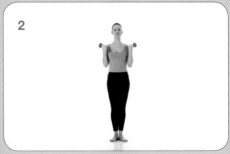

2
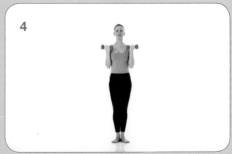

3

4
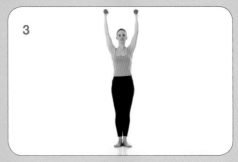

5
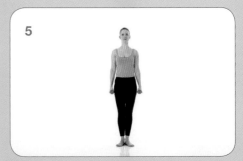

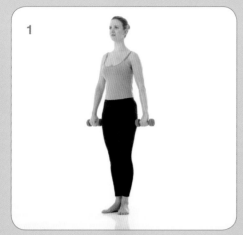

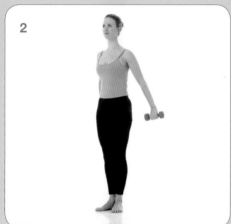

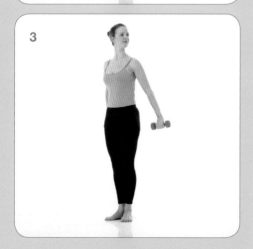

chest expansion

█ beginners

Encourages openness and release across the front of the shoulders while maintaining stability and release in the neck and head.

Equipment Hand-held weights up to approximately 2kg.

starting position

Stand tall on the floor (not on your mat) and lengthen your spine into neutral. Your legs are either parallel and hip-width apart, or connected in Pilates Stance. Hold a weight in each hand and lengthen your arms down by the sides of your body with your palms facing backwards.

Maintain an appropriate level of connection to your centre throughout.

action

● Breathe in and, keeping your arms lengthened and moving only from your shoulder joints, press your arms behind you as far as is possible without disturbing the position of your spine.

● Still breathing in, turn your head to the left, then pass through the centre and turn to the right.

● Breathe out as you return your head to the centre and then lengthen the arms forward, returning them slightly in front of the body.

Repeat up to ten times, alternating the side of the first head turn each time.

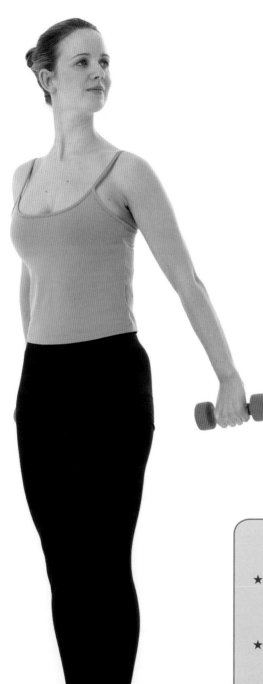

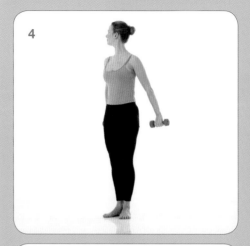

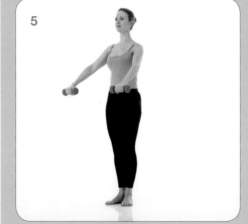

WATCH POINTS

★   Continue to maintain a stable and lengthened, vertical position of your pelvis and spine throughout. Ensure that your upper back does not arch and your ribs do not flare as your press your arms behind you.

★   As you turn your head take care not to tip it back or forwards. It should turn on a central axis as the rest of your spine remains still.

★   Maintain correct wrist alignment: keep your hands and wrists in line with your forearm and avoid rolling your fists away or in towards you.

★   Keep your chest and the front of your shoulders open, especially as you raise your arms upwards.

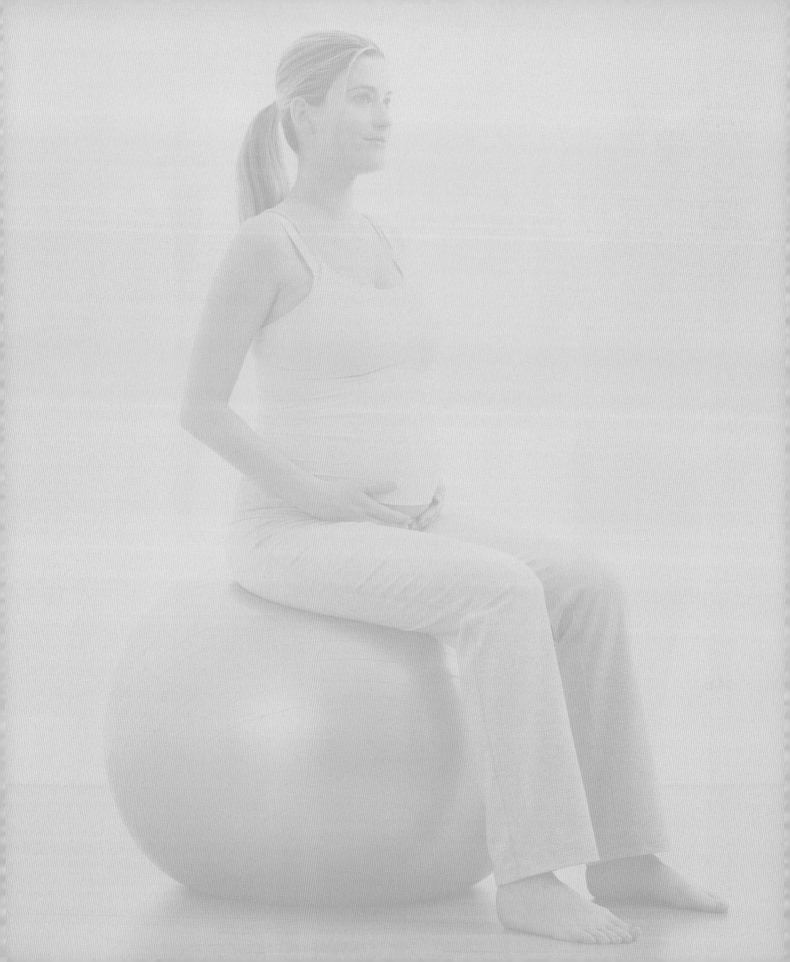

Chapter Six:
Pilates for Health

Pilates can help with a range of common health conditions from poor joint function to mental health issues. The advice in this chapter is by no means meant as a substitute for medical advice, but rather as a guideline for how Pilates can assist with maintaining general health.

Joint health

Many Pilates exercises promote healthy joint function in and around the major joints of the body. In this section we focus individually on the joints of the lower limb, upper limb and the spine. Although problems can occur separately in each of these areas, the cause of many issues lies beyond the area where the symptoms are presenting themselves. For this reason, never discount the benefits of an exercise just because it is not directly working around the area you are concerned with. For instance, improvement in the movement quality of the feet and ankles can have a profound effect on the function and health of the hip joints, which can have a positive influence on the joints of the spine, including the neck and head, which in turn affect the shoulders, elbows and wrists.

In short, improvements made in one area of the body will affect the rest of the body, sometimes subtly, at other times quite dramatically.

There are many types of physiological disorders that affect the health and function of the joints. Conditions such as osteoarthritis are associated with wear and tear of the joint structure. Good joint alignment is one of our key principles and helps to reduce wear and tear on joints. Keeping joints mobile, and strengthening the muscles that support and move them, will also help keep them healthy. Because Pilates exercises are performed with awareness and control they are very safe for people already suffering from such conditions.

Weight management is also a vital part of promoting joint health; carrying too much weight puts excess strain on your joints, especially the knees and hips. Pilates, combined with a healthy balanced diet and cardiovascular activities, offers a realistic and long-term solution to weight management (see Further Information, page 284).

When trying to improve joint function with Pilates exercises, it is important to avoid any movements that you have been advised not to do by your doctor or therapist or that cause you discomfort or pain. With some joint conditions it is inadvisable to perform certain movements. If you are at all unsure whether an exercise is appropriate for you, please check with your doctor or therapist before attempting it.

Generally, thoughtful well-executed movement is the best supplement to any treatment being given for a particular problem. Exercises should be as diverse as possible in order to explore all of the available movement around the joint. Working from varied start positions also ensures that the joint is loaded in different directions, thereby maximising muscular performance.

Each joint has a variety of potential movements. Problems often occur in or around a joint because our everyday activities can cause us to use only a limited part of its potential movement and those movements we do perform are often over-repetitive. Furthermore, the positions we place these joints in for long periods of time are often not 'biomechanically natural' and they therefore become detrimental to the maintenance of good movement and health of the joint. Improvements in movement quality and muscle balance can be enhanced by working through the various ranges of movement with correct form and control. Joint problems arising for other reasons, such as trauma, disease or hereditary causes, may also benefit from this approach to joint health.

Quite simply, when it comes to movement, as with most things in life – use it or lose it!

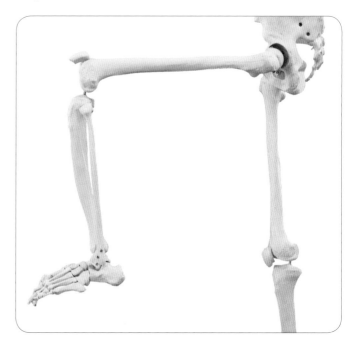

Joints of the lower limb

In this section we look at the hips, knees, ankles and feet. We suggest a range of exercises that utilise the various movements available in each joint and challenge them from a variety of start positions. These exercises can benefit many of the common problems that arise, and working through them will help to

improve specific joints' movements whilst maintaining the dynamic balance of the muscles used to move and control them. Remember, too, that improved function in these lower limb joints may have a positive knock-on effect on the spinal joints.

the hip joint

The hip joint joins the thigh bone (femur) to the pelvis. Its ball-and-socket design is robust enough to support the weight of the body on the legs while still allowing movement in multiple directions. Some of the problems involving the hip joint include: hereditary causes of ball-and-socket development and alignment, trauma to the thigh or hip socket, surgical repair or replacement, degenerative problems caused by wear and tear. More commonly seen, however, are problems arising from the muscles and tendons crossing the joint, most of which are a result of poor use and faulty alignment.

exercises for healthy hips

From the Relaxation Position:
- Leg Slides, Knee Drops and Knee Folds
- Knee Rolls
- Knee Circles
- Zigzags – Lying
- Spine Curls
- Single Leg Stretch

From Side-lying:
- Oyster
- Side Kick Series – Front and Back
- Side Kick Series – Up and Down
- Side Kick Series – Small Circles
- Side Kick Series – Inner Thigh Lift
- Torpedo

From Four-point Kneeling:
- The Cat
- Table Top

From Sitting:
- Zigzags – Sitting

From Prone:
- Prone Beats
- Star

From Standing:
- Roll Downs
- Tennis Ball Rising
- Standing on One Leg
- Standing Leg Press (using the Band)

the knee joint

The knee joint joins the thigh bone (femur) to the bones of the lower leg (tibia and fibula). It is the largest joint in the body with a hinge design that limits its movement potential almost entirely to bending and straightening (flexion and extension). It is a very robust joint as it has to support the entire weight of the body and thigh while still allowing a large range of movement. The most common problems that occur with the joint structure usually result from wear and tear or injury. As the knee lies between the ankle and hip joints, imbalances and dysfunctional use of the muscles and tendons crossing any one of these joints will heighten the risk of injury or damage to the knee. This highlights the importance of improving and maintaining movement quality across the ankles and hips as well as the knees.

exercises for healthy knees

From the Relaxation Position:
- Leg Slides
- Zigzags – Lying
- Single Leg Stretch
- Double Leg Stretch

From Four-point Kneeling:
- Table Top

From Sitting:
- Zigzags – Sitting

From Standing:
- Sliding Down the Wall (using the Big Ball)
- Tennis Ball Rising
- Standing on One Leg
- Standing Leg Press (using the Band)

Leg Slides

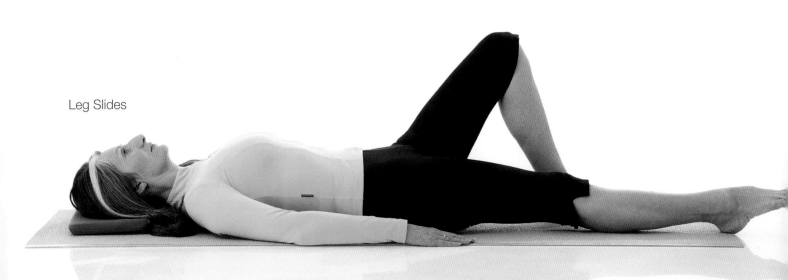

the foot and ankle joints

The joints of the ankles and feet are formed by many individual joints which give rise to an array of different movements; most of them are relatively small and subtle. The largest and most powerful movement is pointing and flexing the foot from the ankle (plantar-flexion and dorsi-flexion). Keeping this joint complex functioning well is important, as the feet are the only point of contact with the ground, performing a vital role in balancing and supporting the rest of the body. Most of the problems arising in this area result from poor alignment and under-use of the structures. Many of our daily activities involve sitting, and when we do actually use our feet they are often crammed into shoes, which limits the full movement and therefore the function of the feet. Given the functional requirements of the feet, it is imperative that exercises are performed in standing as well as other non-weight-bearing positions. Movements that challenge the coordination and control of the intricate movements of the foot can have a positive effect on the function of the ankles, knees, hips and spine.

exercises for healthy feet and ankles

From the Relaxation Position:
- Leg Slides
- Zigzags – Lying
- Ankle Circles
- Creeping Feet

From Sitting:
- Mexican Wave

From Prone:
- Single Leg Kick

From Standing:
- Sliding Down the Wall (using the Big Ball)
- Tennis Ball Rising
- Standing on One Leg

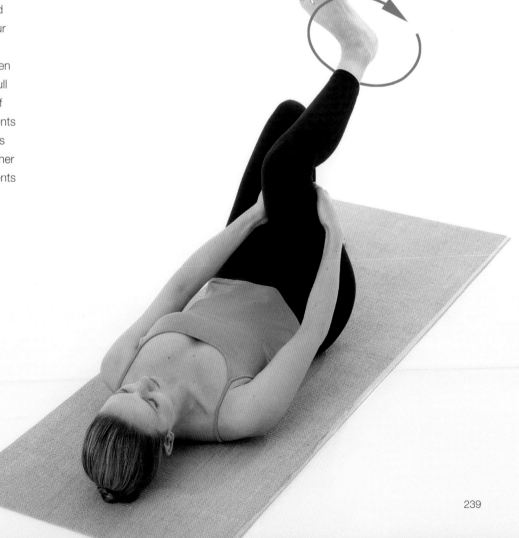

Ankle Circles

Joints of the upper limb

In this section we look at the shoulders, elbows and wrists. Again, we have suggested a range of exercises that employ the various movements available to each joint, challenging them from various start positions. These exercises can help with many of the common problems that arise in and around the upper limb; working through them will help you enhance each joint's range of movement and maintain the dynamic balance of the muscles used to move and control them. The shoulder girdle has an intricate relationship with the spine and torso, in particular the neck. It is therefore important to consider some of the exercises suggested in the spine section (page 242) when looking to improve shoulder function.

the shoulder joints

The shoulder comprises a group of structures that join the upper arm (humerus) to the torso. The main joint of the shoulder joins the upper arm to the shoulder blade (scapula) and allows movements in multiple directions in much the same way as the hip joint does. The shoulder blade should move freely on the back of the ribcage in response to the upper arm and spine. It is joined to the collarbone (clavicle), the other end of which is joined to the breastbone (sternum). The collarbone is able to move up and down above the front of the upper ribcage. The joints between all of these structures should be mobile enough to allow the wide range of motion required in the arms and hands while also remaining strong and stable enough to allow for loaded actions such as lifting, pulling and pushing. Fulfilling these functional requirements demands a complex union between the structures and a fine balance of muscular function, without which the area is susceptible to problems. The degree of mobility within the shoulder and its dependence on good spinal alignment means that the area is vulnerable to the effects of poor posture, which heighten the risk of wear and tear as well as the risk of injury. For this reason it is important to consider the alignment of the upper back and neck in relation to shoulder movement.

exercises for healthy shoulders

From the Relaxation Position:
- Shoulder Drops
- Ribcage Closure
- Ribcage Closure (using the Foam Roller)
- Windows
- Arm Circles
- Curl Ups with Arm Circles (using the Small Ball)
- Flys (using Free Weights)
- Backstroke (using Free Weights)

From Side-lying:
- Bow and Arrow – Lying
- Arm Openings

From Four-point Kneeling:
- The Cat
- Table Top
- Threading the Needle

From Prone:
- Cobra Prep
- Dart

From Standing:
- Dumb Waiter
- Floating Arms

the elbow and wrist joints

The elbow joint comprises three bones: the upper arm (humerus) and the two bones of the forearm (radius and ulna). The wrist joint connects the bones of the forearm to a double row of small bones in the hand (carpals). The joints are similar to the knee and ankle joints in that they primarily allow a hinging action (flexion and extension). However, unlike in the knee and ankle, there is a high degree of rotation available in the forearm between the elbow and wrist. The wrist also allows the hand to hinge from side to side on the forearm (adduct and abduct). Like that of the shoulder, the design of these joints has sacrificed some stability for an increase in mobility. The problems that can occur are often the result of poor movement mechanics. The exposed nature of the joints also leaves them susceptible to injury and strain.

exercises for healthy elbows and wrists

From The Relaxation Position:
- Windows

From Side-lying:
- Bow and Arrow – Lying

From Four-point Kneeling:
- The Cat*
- Threading the Needle*

From Standing:
- Wrist Circles – Standing

* Please note that these exercises may not be suitable for you if you are suffering from strain-related injuries including RSI in the wrists or elbows as they involve weight-bearing on the arms. They are particularly inadvisable if you suffer from carpel tunnel syndrome.

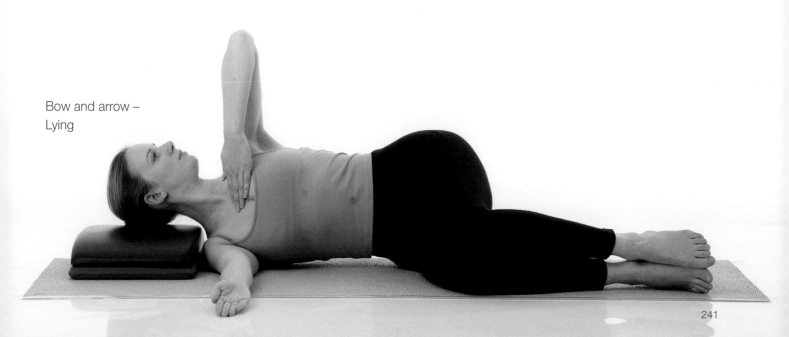

Bow and arrow – Lying

Joints of the spine

The spine consists of twenty-six separate bones and is divided into five regions: cervical, thoracic, lumbar, the sacrum and the coccyx. Each region displays a variety of different characteristics and movement potential.

These bones are connected by a number of ligaments and intervertebral discs. Together they form the vertebral column, also known as the spinal column, which is the central structure upon which the rest of the body is built. It also functions as protection for the spinal cord and provides attachment points for the ribs and the muscles of the back.

Cervical Vertebrae

The cervical region consists of seven bones and forms what we commonly refer to as the neck. These bones allow the neck to bend forwards and backwards (flexion and extension) and from side to side (lateral flexion) as well as turning left and right (rotation). The first two cervical vertebrae relate more to the movement of the head on top of the spine. The first one, also known as 'the atlas', was given its name because it supports the skull (just as Atlas supported the heavens). It primarily allows the head to tip forwards and backwards on the neck. The second cervical vertebra, also called 'the axis', was so named because it acts as a pivot that allows the atlas and the head to rotate on top of the neck.

Thoracic Vertebrae

The thoracic region consists of twelve vertebrae, which start out smaller just like the cervical vertebrae and increase in size until they are similar to the lumbar vertebrae. These twelve bones articulate with one another and with the ribs, forming what we commonly refer to as the torso. The movement available in this area is primarily turning from left to right (rotation) and bending from side to side (lateral flexion). The torso can also bend forwards and backwards (flexion and extension), although the amount of movement is significantly less than is available in the lower back and neck.

Lumbar Vertebrae

The lumbar region or lower back usually consists of five vertebrae (sometimes six or four), which are much larger than the vertebrae above them. This is because the region is subjected to greater loads from the body above and the legs and pelvis below. The movement available in this region is primarily bending backwards and forwards (flexion and extension), with a moderate amount of bending from side to side (lateral flexion). There is next to no rotation available in this region.

Sacrum

The sacrum consists of five fused vertebrae. It is a triangular-shaped bone that joins the last lumbar vertebra to the two halves of the pelvis and the coccyx at the bottom.

Coccyx (Tailbone)

The coccyx usually consists of four fused vertebrae but this can vary between three and five. It is a triangular-shaped bone that offers a small amount of support for the pelvic region.

Given the pivotal role the spine performs it is no wonder that problems in this area can be detrimental to normal functional movement and often cause pain and discomfort. Back pain is one of the most common complaints in western society and is the largest cause of work-related absence. It can affect anyone, regardless of age, but it is more common in people who are between thirty-five and fifty-five years of age. Pain can occur in any region of the back, the most common debilitating back pain usually being reported in the lower back. However, there has been a stark rise in recent years in the instance of neck and shoulder pain, which can become equally incapacitating if left unchecked.

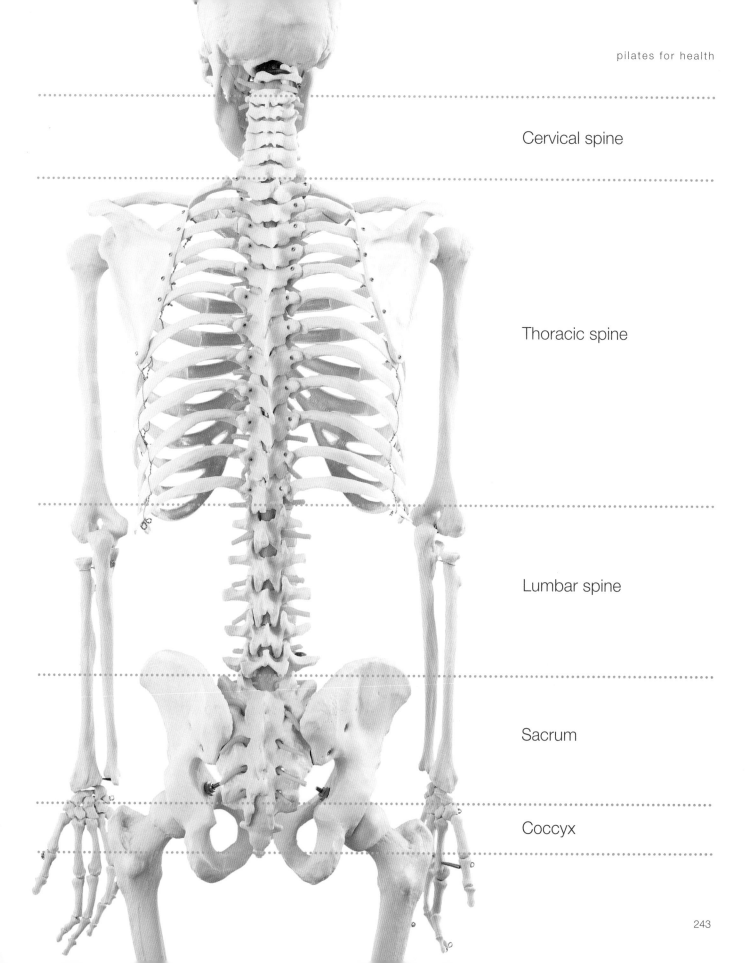

Cervical spine

Thoracic spine

Lumbar spine

Sacrum

Coccyx

the lower back

Lower back pain, sometimes known as lumbago, has been shown in many different studies to affect seven out of ten people at some time during their lives. Symptoms generally occur in between the back of the lower ribs and the top of the legs; they range from general stiffness and aching to more acute and specific pain. Because of the location of and constant demands on the lower back area it's almost impossible to rest effectively during normal daily tasks, so even a moderate level of constant pain and discomfort can become unbearable.

Lower back pain can come on gradually over a long period of time or appear quite suddenly. This is often attributed to a specific event like a fall or awkward bending action. The area is designed to be fairly robust, so unless the event was particularly dramatic the sudden onset of pain is usually the point at which the body can no longer cope with the effects of a sustained period of poor alignment and movement quality. The event triggering the pain response is almost literally 'the straw that broke the camel's back'.

The complex structure of your lower back means that even a small amount of damage or inflammation in that region can cause a large amount of pain and discomfort. In most cases, staying active and continuing carefully with your normal activities will promote healing, thus allowing the back to heal itself. Pain usually lasts between a few days and a few weeks, very rarely longer than six weeks. However, it is important to seek medical advice in persistent or severe cases as an accurate diagnosis of the problem will be necessary. Any treatment for lower back pain will depend largely on the practitioner and their diagnosis of the underlying cause. In the majority of cases doctors and therapists will recommend supplementing any treatment with reconditioning exercises to help tackle the underlying causes. Many actually recommend that their patients take up Pilates exercise. The exercises regularly prescribed by therapists are the same as or very similar to those you will find in this section of the book. Although many of the exercises we have suggested will undoubtedly help in the majority of cases, it is impossible to prescribe a remedial exercise programme without a proper diagnosis, so if in doubt seek medical advice before embarking on any exercise programme.

We have suggested a mixture of exercises that utilise the various movements available to the lower back as well as some that challenge the stability of the area. The selection incorporates a number of different start positions to ensure the muscles in the region get targeted in a variety of ways. Working through these exercises will help you improve the movement quality of the lower back, maintaining the balance of the muscles used to move and control the area. Improved functionality in the lower back is also dependent on achieving release and openness around the hip joints. So as well as the exercises in this section you may want to incorporate some of the exercises suggested in the hip section (page 237)

exercises for a healthy lower back

From the Relaxation Position:
- Leg Slides, Knee Openings and Folds
- Knee Rolls
- Spine Curls
- Hip Rolls
- Curl Ups
- Ribcage Closure
- Ribcage Closure (using the Foam Roller)
- Knee Folds (using the Foam Roller)

From Side-lying:
- Oyster
- Bow and Arrow – Lying
- Arm Openings

From Four-point Kneeling:
- The Cat
- Rest Position
- Threading the Needle
- Table Top
- The Cat (using the Foam Roller)

From Sitting:
- Seated C-Curve
- Waist Twist – Sitting
- Side Reach – Sitting

From Prone:
- Diamond Press
- Dart
- Star

From Standing:
- Roll Downs (using the Band)
- Waist Twist – Standing
- Side Reach – Standing
- Standing Leg Press (using the Band)

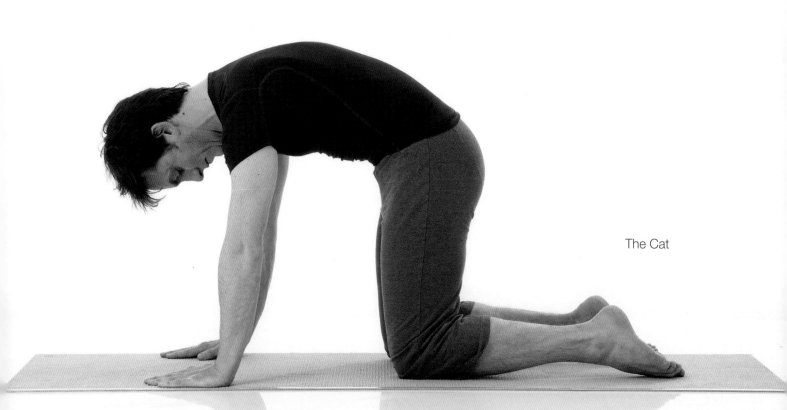

The Cat

the upper back and neck

Pain in the upper back, neck and shoulder regions is also very common, with many people developing symptoms in this region at some time in their lives. Symptoms generally occur anywhere in the upper back and shoulder area, in the neck, and even in and around the head. These usually range from general stiffness and discomfort to more specific acute pain at one or multiple points.

Sustained periods of poor alignment and movement quality account for the vast majority of problems in the neck and shoulders, with symptoms that appear gradually and progressively worsen over time. Symptoms that appear out of the blue are usually the result of a specific event causing strain on the area, like a whiplash injury or a dramatic change in alignment and use. Poor alignment and movement quality will also increase the susceptibility to injuries and strains. As with the lower back, it is important to seek medical advice if symptoms are persistent or severe. In the vast majority of cases, improvements in alignment, posture and movement quality will have a positive effect in reducing or completely removing symptoms of pain and discomfort in the neck and shoulder region.

We have suggested a mixture of exercises that utilise the various movements available to the upper back, neck and head as well as some that challenge the stability of the area by using movements that incorporate the arms and shoulders. The selection includes a number of different start positions to ensure the muscles in the region get targeted in a variety of ways. Working through these exercises will help you improve the movement quality of the whole area, maintaining the dynamic balance of the muscles used to move and control it. Improvements in and around the upper back and neck are largely dependent on achieving release and openness around the shoulders. So, as well as the exercises in this section, you should incorporate some of the exercises suggested in the shoulder section (page 240).

exercises for a healthy upper back and neck

From the Relaxation Position:
- Chin Tucks and Neck Rolls
- Nose Circles (using the Small Ball)
- Spine Curls
- Curl Ups
- Curl Ups with Arm Circles (using the Small Ball)
- Ribcage Closure
- Ribcage Closure (using the Foam Roller)
- Windows
- Flys (using Free Weights)
- Backstroke (using Free Weights)

From Side-lying:
- Bow and Arrow – Lying
- Arm Openings

From Four-point Kneeling:
- The Cat
- Rest Position
- Threading the Needle
- Table Top
- The Cat (using the Foam Roller)
- Diamond Press (using the Big Ball)

From Sitting:
- Seated C-Curve
- Waist Twist – Sitting
- Side Reach – Sitting

From Prone:
- Diamond Press
- Dart
- Star

From Standing:
- Roll Downs (using the Band)
- Waist Twist – Standing
- Side Reach – Standing
- Standing Leg Press (using the Band)

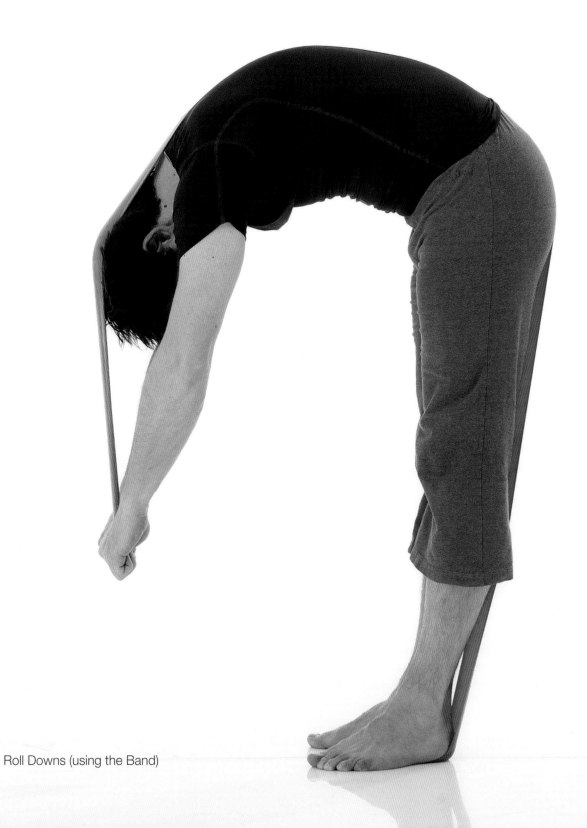

Roll Downs (using the Band)

Bone health

Your bone health is determined by a number of factors: genetic make-up, hormonal status, nutrition, mineral and vitamin content and the amount of stress the bone is put under. Bones are thicker and stronger when they are stressed, as stress produces electrical effects in the bone, which in turn encourage bone growth. If there is no stress, the bone will be less dense and weaker. Recent research has shown that regular weight-bearing exercise can help improve bone health and the earlier we start weight training, the better, even in our teens, as we are then laying good foundations for the future.

Osteoporosis is a skeletal disease, which involves the gradual and painless loss of bone, increasing the fragility of bones and making them prone to fracture. One in two women and one in five men over the age of fifty in the UK will break a bone as the result of osteoporosis. The World Health Organisation suggested in 1999 that this problem was reaching epidemic proportions throughout the world. Men and young people can be affected by osteoporosis but it is most common in post-menopausal women. This is because there is rapid bone loss in the years immediately following the menopause.

Although bone looks very solid, in fact it is full of holes rather like coral. It has a thick outer shell of cortical bone and a honeycomb inner mesh of tiny struts of trabecular bone. With osteoporosis or osteopenia, which is the precursor to osteoporosis, some of these struts become thin and may break. Having osteoporosis does not automatically mean that your bones will break, but it does mean that you are at a greater risk of fracture. These fractures may occur in different parts of the body but are most common at the wrist, hip and spine. Often the first indication that a person has low bone density is a fracture of the wrist. This is because we normally react to a fall by putting out our arms. While the disease itself does not cause any pain, bone fractures are painful and can lead to other health problems.

Your bone mineral density can be assessed by a quick pain-free procedure called a dual energy X-ray absorptiometry Scan. After this you will be given a T-score, which indicates how much your bone density differs from that of a normal young adult. Usually osteoporosis is treated with a combination of drugs and lifestyle changes, including nutrition and exercise advice. Weight-bearing exercise is recommended and, if you are at risk of fracture, a falls-prevention programme.

Pilates can help maintain and improve bone health and help to prevent falls. The focus on good posture, core stability, balance and coordination is very beneficial. Many of the exercises in this book are weight-bearing – using the body's own weight against gravity. You will also find exercises using light free weights and resistance. Furthermore, as Pilates strengthens your muscles, it will also help to improve bone density as the muscles then pull on the bones, which can in turn stimulate bone growth.

However, if you have already been diagnosed with osteopenia or osteoporosis, you will need to consult your medical practitioner before embarking on a Pilates programme and you may need to adapt your programme accordingly. Depending on the degree and site of bone loss, you may be advised to avoid certain movements whilst exercising.

As a general rule any exercise which involves flexion of the spine is contraindicated, so avoid exercises such as Curl Ups, The Hundred, Single Leg Stretch, Double Leg Stretch, Roll Downs, Roll Backs and Spine Curls.

Similarly, your practitioner may advise against exercise that involves 'loaded' rotation or 'loaded' side flexion: Hip Rolls with the feet off the floor, Mermaid and The Saw (which is both flexion and rotation) fall into this category. Normally gentle spinal rotation, such as Arm Openings and Waist Twist, and gentle side flexion, such as Side Reach, are still permitted, but check with your practitioner first.

Having both legs lifted from the floor (as, for example, in Torpedo or Swimming) may put too much pressure on the spine so it is best avoided. If you have osteoporosis in your hip, avoid adducting the leg (bringing it across the mid-line of the body) or medially rotating the legs, as in Knee Rolls.

Try to include lots of back extension exercises, such as Diamond Press, Dart, Cobra prep and Star, in your workouts.

exercises for improving bone health

Note: please consult your medical practitioner if you have been diagnosed with osteoporosis. Exercises that help improve awareness and control of neutral spine are very beneficial, as are those that include hinging from the hips, such as Pilates Squats.

- Leg Slides
- Knee Openings
- Knee Folds – Single
- Ribcage Closure
- Bow and Arrow – Lying
- Oyster
- Dart
- Diamond Press
- Cobra Prep
- Star
- Single Leg Kick
- Table Top
- Rest Position
- Biceps Press (using Free Weights)
- Chest Expansion (using Free Weights)

By a supporting wall:

- Tennis Ball Rising
- Standing on One Leg
- Sliding Down the Wall (using the Big Ball)
- Waist Twist – Standing
- Side Reach – Standing
- Pilates Squats

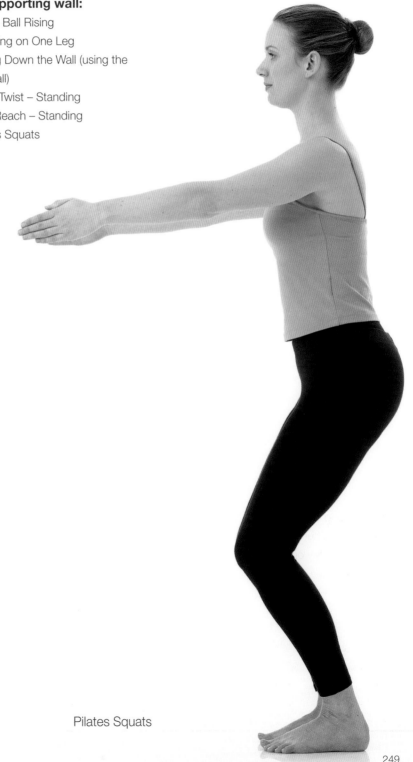

Pilates Squats

Heart health

Although Pilates is a fabulous mind-and-body conditioning method, it is not a cardiovascular workout. For your total health and wellbeing you will need to add some aerobic activities to your fitness regime in addition to your Pilates practice.

In January 2007, the American College of Sports Medicine and the American Heart Association issued a report stating that to provide and maintain health, all healthy adults aged between eighteen and sixty-five need moderate-intensity aerobic (endurance) physical activity for either a minimum of thirty minutes on five days each week, or more vigorous-intensity aerobic physical activity for a minimum of twenty minutes on three days a week. They also advise adding eight to ten strength-training exercises (with eight to twelve repetitions of each exercise) per week. Regular Pilates practice will contribute to this. Moderate-intensity physical activity means working hard enough to raise your heart rate and break into a sweat, yet still be able to carry on a conversation.

If weight loss is your goal or if you wish to maintain your weight, sixty to ninety minutes of physical activity may be necessary. The thirty-minute recommendation is for the average healthy adult to maintain health and reduce risk of chronic disease.

The guidelines for adults over sixty-five (or adults with chronic conditions such as arthritis) are either moderately intense aerobic exercise for thirty minutes a day, five days per week, or vigorously intense aerobic exercises twenty minutes a day, three days per week. It is also advised that you add eight to ten strength-training exercises (with ten to fifteen repetitions of each exercise) two or three times per week. Follow strength training with flexibility work. And, if you are at risk of falling, perform balance exercises. Once again, regular Pilates practice will contribute to these.

Cardiovascular Choices

You can choose from a multitude of activities: some require gym membership, others joining a class, but there are also plenty of 'free' outdoor activities as well:

* Brisk walking
* Jogging
* Walking on an incline
* Running
* Hiking
* Cycling
* Cross-country running
* Skiing
* Aerobic dance
* Skipping
* Rowing
* Stair climbing
* Swimming
* Skating
* Rebounding

To keep yourself motivated, choose an activity that you enjoy. And be sure to remember everything that you have learnt in your Pilates practice. Chapter Seven provides specific guidelines on how to apply your Pilates technique to various gym activities, sports and hobbies.

The Problem of Obesity

Recent years have seen an alarming growth in the number of people classified as obese. This problem is affecting so many countries in the western world that it has become an international health concern. Being overweight, obese or morbidly obese significantly increases the risk of developing many diseases such as heart disease, diabetes, hypertension, osteoarthritis and more.

An individual is considered obese when their body mass index (BMI) measures 30 or higher (see below), and morbidly obese when they have a BMI of 40 or higher.

The adoption of a healthy and active lifestyle and healthy eating habits are central to solving the problem, for both adults and children. If you think you may be obese or if you feel that have a lot of weight to lose, please contact your local GP who can offer you advice and support. With your doctor's permission, you may be able to try some of the gentle movements in the Fundamentals and Beginners' Programme. You may also like to refer to the book *Pilates for Weight Loss* (see Further Information, page 284). As you gain more confidence in your ability to move, you will gradually be able to increase your overall levels of activity.

Balancing mind and body

Mental health

As Pilates is a complete mind-body approach we also look at how it can improve the health of our minds. Mental health is still often a taboo subject. However, mental issues affect us all in one way or another, from varying degrees of stress or anxiety to more serious conditions. Pilates helps us to keep our minds in tip-top condition as well as supplementing the recovery from physical or mental stress.

First, it can help balance out the negative effects our state of mind can have on our body. It has often been said that our bodies are the graveyard of human emotions. How often do we refer to someone or something that causes us stress as 'a pain in the neck'? The emotions of love and sadness can manifest themselves physically in a dramatic way; we quite literally feel our emotions and this can take its toll on our body. Our physical demeanour can reflect our state of mind; how we carry ourselves says a lot about how we feel. Pilates is the perfect way to rebalance the body, helping undo the physical tension that the mind can cause.

Second, Pilates can balance out the negative effects our body can have on our emotional state. Just as the mind influences the body, the body also influences the mind. If we feel well physically, we generally feel better mentally. Poor posture, discomfort and pain can have a negative impact on our state of mind. Simply improving the posture and ease of movement can be emotionally uplifting, improving self-esteem and self-image. Another way that Pilates exercises can positively influence our minds is through the intense focus and concentration they demand in the control and precision of the movements involved. Focusing intently on controlling the body, helps channel the mind away from the thoughts that normally occupy it, many of which can cause stress and anxiety.

Managing neurological disorders

As well as helping maintain the balance of health in mind and body, Pilates can also help support the recovery and management of many neurological conditions that affect the control and coordination of movement. Working with thoughtful movement will have a positive training effect on the central nervous system, which connects our mind and body. Many physical therapies seek to influence the central nervous system through movement function. Pilates can really help supplement any treatment being given by a trained therapist. If you suffer from any kind of neurological disorder, ask your medical practitioner whether they feel Pilates exercises would complement the treatment they are giving.

exercises to balance mind and body

The very nature of all Pilates exercise helps balance the mind and body. However, this selection of exercises is particularly helpful in releasing mental stress and the physical tension it can lead to. Try them the next time you feel your thoughts weighing you down.

- Shoulder Drops
- Ribcage Closure
- Leg Slides and Knee Circles
- Spine Curls

- Hip Rolls
- Waist Twist – Sitting
- Side Reach – Sitting

- Cobra Prep
- The Cat
- Rest Position

Antenatal pilates

Pregnancy is a perfectly normal state, not an illness. Yet as a pregnant woman your exercise needs will change literally month by month and you will need to adapt your exercise routine accordingly. The many benefits Pilates has to offer during pregnancy are summarised below.

● It teaches you body awareness.

● It helps to improve posture which in turn reduces the strain on joints.

● It can help ensure that your body's systems (circulatory, lymphatic, respiratory, digestive) are all functioning efficiently.

● It can teach relaxation and breathing skills, which will be invaluable throughout the pregnancy and also during the birth itself.

● By improving pelvic stability, Pilates may help to prevent pelvic girdle pain. Hormonal changes in the body affect your ligaments (which join bone to bone): they soften to allow the pelvis to expand during the birth itself. This means, however, that many of your joints may become unstable, in particular the sacroiliac and symphysis pubis joints.

● The additional weight of the breasts and laxity of the ligaments often cause shoulder and neck problems. By improving upper-body posture and movement, Pilates can be instrumental in helping to reduce these problems.

● The deep core muscles strengthened by Pilates exercises will help support the growing weight of the baby, and your spine, by creating a natural girdle of strength. This may be very helpful in reducing back pain.

● As the pregnancy progresses, there is a shift in your centre of gravity. This, combined with the effect of the hormones on spatial awareness, can result in changes to balance and coordination.

● Many foot, ankle and knee problems start during pregnancy because of the extra weight being carried as well as the laxity of the ligaments. (See pages 238–239 for relevant exercises, but please note the advice given below on safe practice for each trimester.) Many of the foot exercises may be done seated.

● Pilates can help prepare the pelvic floor to carry increased weight, for the birth itself and for postnatal recovery.

● It can help to prepare you for the rigours of labour, which is what it says it is – extremely hard work!

All pregnant mothers, regardless of levels of fitness, should seek medical approval before embarking on a new exercise regime. It is also advisable to check with your medical practitioner at regular intervals during the pregnancy that it is still safe for you to exercise. We recommend that you stop exercising between weeks eight and fourteen of the pregnancy unless you are under specialist guidance. If you're new to Pilates, find a suitably qualified Pilates teacher (see Further Information, page 284).

Many of our clients have benefited from gentle Pilates exercise through their first trimester but this is under close supervision. With this in mind we have focused here on exercises for second and third trimesters.

Second Trimester (thirteen to twenty-six weeks)

Whilst our goal will be to keep your abdominals strong, we will be doing this with pelvic-stability-style exercises rather than exercises which involve trunk flexion such as Curl Ups, Single Leg Stretch or The Hundred. This is because, as the pregnancy progresses, your abdominals separate to allow room for the baby and uterus to grow. It is inadvisable to strengthen these muscles in a shortened position until they have drawn back together after the birth. Please do not be tempted to do The Hundred, Double Leg Stretch, or similar exercises, with the head down as this would place an enormous strain on your lower back.

The exercises below will help to keep your body supple and flexible, but you should avoid over-stretching as your joints will be prone to instability. Also avoid exercises that put pressure on the pubic bone (Spine Stretch Forward and The Saw).

From about sixteen weeks on you need to aware of a condition called supine hypotensive syndrome, which results in dizziness and low blood pressure when lying on your back, caused by the weight of the uterus compressing the vena cava (the largest vein in the trunk) and so restricting blood flow to the heart. Some practitioners advise their patients not to exercise lying on their backs at all during the last two trimesters of pregnancy. You will need to consult your individual practitioner.

Some of our beginners' exercises, which are normally done lying on the mat, may be adapted to a seated or standing position (see below). For example, you could use the Starting Position as described in Sliding Down the Wall (page 218).

If you do decide to include a few supine exercises, please remember to change position after three minutes and to keep your limbs moving whilst lying on your back. If you do feel nauseous or dizzy, turn over onto your left side.

Choose exercises that keep your body symmetrical and avoid single leg weight bearing. We make use of the Big Ball (used during labour in some hospitals) in the workouts. Take extra care when moving from one exercise to the next and follow your natural breathing rhythm.

As abdominal hollowing becomes a thing of the past, think of the cue to 'zip up from the pelvic floor and lift your bump' or 'zip and hug the baby'. You may continue with prone exercises until it becomes uncomfortable or up to twenty-four weeks.

second trimester workout

- Sliding Down the Wall (using the Big Ball)
- Leg Slides (if supine permitted)
- Spine Curls (small curls only)
- The Pelvic Elevator
- The Emergency Stop
- Bow and Arrow – Sitting
- Side Reach – Sitting
- The Cat

- Table Top (keep hands and feet in contact with the mat)
- Single Knee Folds (if supine permitted)
- Hip Rolls – feet down
- Arm Openings (as the bump grows use an extra pillow to support it)
- Oyster (avoid if you have pelvic girdle pain)
- Side-lying Legs Circles (bend your underneath leg and place a pillow under your bump)

- Windows (if supine permitted)
- Diamond Press (using the Big Ball).
- Arm Circles Back Over the Big Ball
- Foot Exercises (these may be done seated)
- Tennis Ball Rising
- Pilates Squats

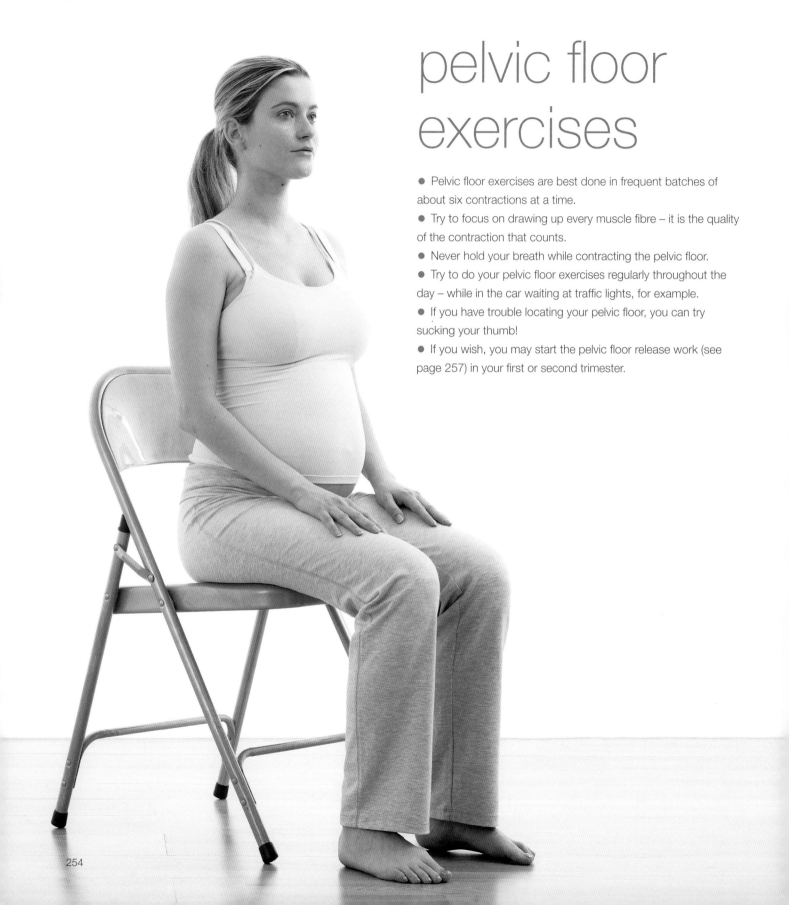

pelvic floor exercises

● Pelvic floor exercises are best done in frequent batches of about six contractions at a time.

● Try to focus on drawing up every muscle fibre – it is the quality of the contraction that counts.

● Never hold your breath while contracting the pelvic floor.

● Try to do your pelvic floor exercises regularly throughout the day – while in the car waiting at traffic lights, for example.

● If you have trouble locating your pelvic floor, you can try sucking your thumb!

● If you wish, you may start the pelvic floor release work (see page 257) in your first or second trimester.

the pelvic elevator

Helps improve pelvic floor awareness, control and tone.

starting position

Sit upright on a chair. Place your feet on the floor, either hip-width apart or connecting your inner thighs together. Make sure that your weight is even on both sitting bones and that your spine is lengthened in neutral.

Imagine that your pelvic floor is a lift in a building. This exercise requires you to take the 'lift' up to different floors of the building – three floors to be precise.

preparation

● Breathe wide into your ribs and lengthen your spine.
● Breathe out as you visualise gently sliding the doors of the lift shut, and then taking the lift to the first floor of the building. As if you are zipping from the back to the front of your pelvic floor region, first lift from your back passage as if trying to prevent yourself from passing wind, then bring this feeling forward towards your pubic bone as if trying to stop yourself from passing water. Continue gently to draw these muscles up inside.
● Breathe in and focus on keeping the lift on the first floor with the doors shut. This will help you gently to maintain the connection of your pelvic floor muscles.

● Breathe out as you slowly take the lift up, a little higher to the second floor. Engage your pelvic floor muscles slightly more.
● Breathe in and hold the lift on the second floor.
● Breathe out as you take the lift to the third floor. Gently engage your pelvic floor muscles even more, but avoid over-gripping this area.
● Breathe in as you hold the lift on the third floor
● Breathe out as you slowly lower the lift back down, floor by floor until your reach the ground floor and allow the doors to slide open. Literally, you will gradually release your pelvic floor with control and eventually release this area completely. Repeat up to five times.

WATCH POINTS

★ Ensure that you do not pull up or in too hard. It is very important that you do not force this pelvic floor action or grip.

★ Make sure that you keep your buttock muscles relaxed. Your pelvis remains still throughout: the action of the 'lift' is purely internal.

★ Keep your chest and the front of your shoulders open and avoid any tension in your neck area.

★ Continue to breathe fully throughout; it is very important not to hold your breath.

the emergency stop

Stress incontinence is surprisingly common. The following exercise will help you to cope with emergencies such as when coughing or sneezing.

● Simply lift the whole of the pelvic floor, tightening it all quickly as if in an emergency. Hold for about five seconds, then release. Repeat up to five times.

Third Trimester (twenty-seven to forty weeks)

The advice given above for the second trimester is also relevant during this later stage of your pregnancy. In addition to the pelvic floor exercises on page 255, you should start to include exercises that teach you how to relax your pelvic floor in readiness for the delivery of your baby. Include plenty of squatting exercises as these help to open the pelvic outlet.

Four-point Kneeling is a wonderful position in these later stages of pregnancy as it helps position the baby for the birth.

Advice on the Workout

There are a lot of position changes in this workout as you will probably become uncomfortable in one position quite quickly. As before, take your time to change position. If you have been lying, always roll slowly onto your side before getting up from the floor.

Remember that you may adapt some of the beginners' exercises to be done in seated or standing by a wall.

third trimester workout

- Pilates Squats
- The Flower
- Pelvic Rocking in Four-point Kneeling
- Dumb Waiter – Sitting
- Chest Expansion – Sitting (no weights)
- Waist Twist – Sitting
- Shoulder Drops (if supine permitted)
- Spine Curls (small curls only)
- Bow and Arrow – Lying (extra pillow supporting bump)
- Ribcage Closure (stand by the wall if supine not permitted)
- Pelvic Elevator (include the basement!)
- Feet Exercises – Sitting
- Arm Circles Back Over the Big Ball
- Side Reach – Sitting
- Zigzags – Sitting
- Pilates Squats (using Big Ball)
- Sliding Down the Wall (using Big Ball)

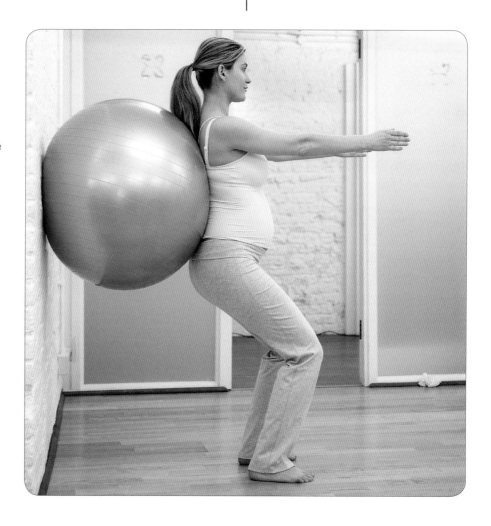

pelvic floor release exercises

It is very important that you allow your mouth to remain soft and released as you do these exercises. If you like, you may blow softly through your mouth as you release the pelvic floor. It helps to blow against your hand.

the flower

Helps you learn how to control and release the pelvic floor muscles.

starting position

Either align yourself correctly in the Four-point Kneeling Position, or sit upright on a chair.

preparation

- Breathe in and prepare your body.
- Breathe out as you gather together and gradually draw up the muscles of your pelvic floor inside you; imagining a flower closing.
- Breathe in and gently hold the flower closed.
- Breathe out as you slowly allow the flower to open completely.
- Breathe in and ever so slightly close the flower, to return the pelvic floor to its normal tone.

Repeat up to five times.

WATCH POINTS

★ Ensure that your pelvis remains still throughout: the subtle close and release of the flower is purely internal. Make sure that you keep your buttock muscles relaxed.

★ Continue to breathe fully throughout – it is very important not to hold your breath.

★ Keep your chest and the front of your shoulders open and avoid any tension in your neck area.

the pelvic elevator – release

Follow the first seven action points for the Pelvic Elevator (page 255), but on your next out-breath release the 'lift' down to the basement. Then breathe in and gently bring the lift back up to the ground floor.

Postnatal

Normally when we refer to the postnatal period, we mean the six weeks following the birth. However, it takes the body at least nine months to recover fully from pregnancy, even longer if you are still breastfeeding. So perhaps it is more appropriate to think of nine months pregnant, nine months in postnatal recovery.

Your midwife/medical practitioner will need to give you the go-ahead to start exercising again. Much will depend on the length and nature of your labour and the type of delivery you had. No two births are the same.

We described how the abdominals separate during pregnancy to allow the baby to grow. Sometimes the abdominals do not draw back together sufficiently and this may have an impact on how well these muscles can support the spine. This is called a diastasis recti and your medical or fitness professional should be able to check if this affects you. Any separation of more than two fingers' width or any sign of the abdominals doming when you perform a Curl Up, say, will mean that you should avoid trunk flexion and work to improve your pelvic stability and abdominal strength with a gentle progressive programme (see below).

Among our goals over the next few months are:
- to strengthen your pelvic floor muscles;
- to work on your pelvic and lumbar stability;
- to strengthen your deep abdominals progressively to help correct the separation of the abdominals;
- to help improve your upper body movement and posture to counter the effects of breast- or bottle-feeding and infant care;
- to help you relax.

Urinary stress and urge incontinence are very common both during pregnancy and postnatally. After all, the baby has been bouncing up and down on your pelvic floor for the last few months. The birthing process may also have damaged the pelvic floor. Sometimes, you need extra help with locating and strengthening your pelvic floor. If you feel that you need help, please ask your medical practitioner to refer you to a women's health physiotherapist (see Further Information, page 284).

postnatal workout

- Pelvic Floor Exercises,* slow and fast (pages 255–257). You can practise engaging your pelvic floor and abdominal hollowing in a variety of positions:
- Sitting
- Relaxation Position
- Side-lying
- Prone
- Standing – also with the legs further apart, which makes it more challenging

- Pilates Stance
- Basic Pelvic Stability exercises
- Leg Slides*
- Knee Openings*

- Single Knee Folds*
- Chin Tucks and Neck Rolls
- Shoulder Drops
- Spine Curls
- Ribcage Closure
- Hip Rolls – Feet down
- Arm Openings
- Star
- Diamond Press
- Dart
- The Cat
- Rest Position
- Zigzags – Lying
- Side Reach – Standing
- Dumb Waiter (with neck turn)

- Chest Expansion (no weights)
- Pilates Stance

Reintroduce Curl Ups only when the diastasis is less than two fingers' width and there is no sign of the abdominals doming.

* If you do have stress incontinence, please practise pelvic floor contractions regularly throughout the day. Do six repetitions, held for ten seconds, ten times a day (no more than this or you risk fatiguing the muscles).

Menopause and post-menopause

There is no greater preparation for later life than regular Pilates practice. Your joints and bones will be healthy, your spine flexible and strong. Middle-age spread is not inevitable; it may not be quite so easy to keep your body toned, but if you can do three hours of Pilates every week, the results will be clearly evident. There is nothing quite as ageing as poor posture, which is why the workout below focuses on improving posture.

You will still need to add some cardiovascular work into your exercise programme. Brisk walking and swimming are excellent options. Try to manage your weight, as this will have an impact on the health of your joints and also your overall health. Be alert, in particular, for any extra weight gain around the waist, as extra fat stored in this area has been linked with many health problems.

Pilates, combined with a healthy balanced diet and regular aerobic exercise, will help you to keep your weight under control and will also assist in reducing some of the more unpleasant symptoms of the menopause.

As well as helping to reduce stress, Pilates can also keep your brain active. Each time you learn a new exercise, you are acquiring new movement skills, challenging your coordination and learning choreography.

As we grow older, it becomes even more important to work on the pelvic floor muscles. A prolapsed uterus is very common in post-menopausal women. The pelvic floor exercises described in the postnatal section opposite will be appropriate for you, but please consult your medical practitioner if you experience any unusual sensation or bulging in the pelvic floor area.

There is no upper age limit to doing Pilates. We have clients well into their nineties still enjoying classes!

menopause workout

From the Relaxation Position:
- Shoulder Drops
- Chin Tucks and Neck Rolls
- Knee Circles
- Spine Curls
- Hip Rolls – feet down
- Knee Rolls

From Side-lying:
- Oyster
- Arm Openings

From Prone:
- Diamond Press
- Dart
- Cobra Prep

From Four-point Kneeling:
- The Cat
- Table Top (keep your feet down and your arms still)
- Rest Position

From Standing:
- Feet Exercises
- Wrist Circles
- The Pelvic Elevator
- The Emergency Stop
- Tennis Ball Rising
- Side Reach – Standing
- Waist Twist – Standing
- Pilates Squats
- Standing on One Leg (by a supporting wall)

Chapter Seven: Pilates for Work and Play

sedentary lifestyle

These days much of our life can be spent doing very little physically, both at work and at leisure. The digital revolution has enabled us to work and play from a chair with no more effort required than a few taps of our fingers. The negative effects sedentary living has on our health and longevity have been widely publicised over recent years. However, many of us dismiss these long-term effects on the premise that 'it won't happen to me!' Less well known is the fact that a sedentary lifestyle also has grave implications for the musculoskeletal system. These can affect us in the short term as well as the long term in the form of pain and discomfort, which can reduce our quality of living and even affect our mental health. Even if you do nothing else (and we suggest that you do!), performing a few simple Pilates exercises a day can help keep the aches and pains at bay.

When you have to sit still for long periods at a time it is important to consider your alignment. Breaking up periods of sitting with some of the simple exercises we have suggested can make a world of difference to your comfort levels.

Work

Many of us have jobs that involve sitting all day at a desk. This is not what our bodies were designed for and as a result often, by lunchtime, you are feeling the strain. A well-designed workstation is vital and should be the first thing you look at if you are starting to develop pain or discomfort. Being more aware of your posture and taking short breaks from sitting every hour or so will make a big difference. It is highly advantageous to fill those breaks with some of the simple exercises suggested to help rebalance the body and boost your mental energy.

Are you sitting comfortably?

Sit tall on your chair. Have both feet firmly grounded on the floor, hip-width apart and parallel. The idea is for the knees to be bent at an angle of about ninety degrees, the heels lined up with the back of the knees. You may need to place your feet on a low platform (or a couple of large books) to achieve this.

Check that your weight is evenly balanced in the centre of both sitting bones. We are aiming for an elongated S-shape for the spine, not a collapsed C-shape. So check that you have a gentle hollow in the lower back (lumbar lordosis). Avoid rolling back onto your coccyx, which would take you into a slouched C-shape. Similarly avoid rolling too far forwards towards your pubic bone as this would cause the lower back to over-arch. Instead lengthen up through the whole spine so that its natural curves are retained. It is not easy to maintain this elongated S-shape. Regular Pilates practice will make it much easier as your deep postural muscles are strengthened. In the meantime, if it is more comfortable, you may place a small support in the lumbar curve (a rolled-up towel or even a Small Ball inflated to about 25 per cent or whatever is comfortable).

Allow your ribcage to relax and be positioned directly above the pelvis, neither swaying backwards nor slumping forwards. Feel your shoulder blades wide in the upper back and your collarbones open in the front of the chest. Soften your breastbone. Lengthen your neck and allow your head to balance freely on top of the spine.

If you have space you can sit on a Big Ball instead of a chair for short spells during the day. Sitting correctly on the Ball will help you re-establish the dynamic stability needed to maintain good posture throughout the day. Its natural instability means that your core stability muscles have to work harder to keep you upright and balanced. Its bounciness also encourages you to stay mobile and active. We do not recommend that you spend all day on the Ball; shorter periods of time spent focusing on maintaining good posture are very beneficial. However, if you spend too long on the Ball, your body will tire and your focus will lapse, leaving you in a very awkward position or even on the floor! Slouching whilst on the Ball is a lot worse than doing so on a chair as the chair will at least provide a level of support.

Recreation

When we get home often the first thing we want to do is sit back in our favourite chair and put our feet up. Once there we will reach for any number of things to entertain ourselves: the latest book, the remote control, a laptop computer, a games console, sewing or knitting. All have one thing in common – sitting. However, the sitting element disregards our bodies' need to move. Supplementing these sedentary activities with some active ones is always advisable. So remember, take a break from time to time and get your body moving.

exercises for a sedentary lifestyle

Seated

Waist Twist – Sitting
Side Reach – Sitting
Dumb Waiter
Bow and Arrow
Floating Arms
Ankle Circles
Wrist Circles
Mexican Wave
Neck Rolls
Zigzags – Sitting

Standing

Tennis Ball Rising
Pilates Squats
Chest Expansion
Sliding Down the Wall
Roll Downs

Travel

Travelling, like other sedentary activities, puts the body under pressure. The relative inactivity along with brief periods of lugging heavy bags around can heighten the risk of stresses and strains too. Another much publicised issue is deep vein thrombosis (DVT), which has become associated with flying, especially long-haul flights. There is a variety of reasons why you may be more at risk of developing DVT during air travel, but the key factor is immobility. However, sitting still for too long is not restricted to flying – you can develop DVT during any long-distance travel by train or car, or even while watching a movie!

To help minimise this risk, try to stay mobile and avoid sitting still for more than two hours at a time. Do the exercises recommended above before, during and after your journey to keep your joints released and your circulatory system functioning well.

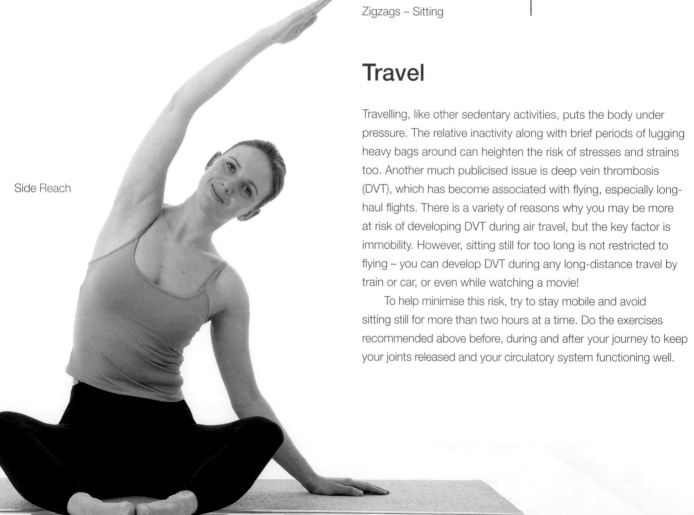

Side Reach

active lifestyle

Just as under-use of the body can be detrimental, excessive or repetitive physical activity can also have negative implications. Like everything in life it is about striking a balance. If the objectives of your physical activity are primarily improved health and recreation, moderation is the key to keeping your body's systems in good balance, helping you feel and perform well. If, however, your physical activities are part of your job or are more serious and competitive than light-hearted recreation, the balance often tips in favour of performance over healthy use of the body. Pilates is an ideal way to offset the negative effects of over-use, helping you readdress the balance and perform to the best of your ability. It can even enhance your performance by making your movements more efficient. Pilates can also help you recover from injuries by supplementing any treatment you are receiving.

Whether you have to perform physically as part of your job or in your recreational activities, Pilates will help improve your performance.

Please note: We are not offering suggestions for rehabilitation for the problems that can occur with these various activities, but we hope that the suggested exercises and advice will help keep you injury-free and enhance your enjoyment and ability to perform them. If you do have an injury as a result of a physical activity,

first get it properly diagnosed and treated by a professional therapist or doctor and then refer to the section on joint health (page 236) for suggestions on supplementing any treatment you are receiving.

Manual Work

Although physical challenge is generally considered a good thing for our bodies, the repetitive nature of manual work means the body is being challenged in the same way day in, day out. This can take its toll just as much as sitting at a desk all day. The biggest cause of problems is undoubtedly over-use and strains due to poor movement technique. Even if you are highly skilled in the movements you have to perform daily, injuries can still occur as bad technique can creep in when you are tired or your concentration lapses. Pilates can help with this by improving self-awareness, posture, coordination and control. Try some of the key exercise suggestions sporadically throughout your working day to help keep the body and mind alert.

From a practical perspective we suggest that you perform all of these exercises either standing or sitting when in the work place.

exercises for an active lifestyle

Back and neck
- Neck Rolls*
- Side Bends – Standing
- Waist Twists – Standing
- Bow and Arrow – Sitting#
- Seated C-Curve#
- Diamond Press*
- Curl Ups*
- Oblique Curl Ups*

Shoulders and arms
- Floating Arms
- Ribcage Closure*
- Arm Circles*
- Bicep Curl and Press
- Windows*

Hips and legs
- Tennis Ball Rising
- Pilates Squats
- Single Leg Kick*

- Zigzags – Sitting#
- Side Kick Series – Front and Back*

* These exercises are normally performed from lying on the mat; try to reproduce the same movement from a standing position and use a wall to simulate the floor.

These seated exercises may also be performed from a chair rather than the floor.

Housework and DIY

The specific physical demands of many household chores can certainly take their toll on our bodies if not performed with good technique. The problem is no one ever sits us down to teach us the best way to vacuum the house or how to reach, bend and twist into awkward spaces when cleaning, let alone how to paint a ceiling! Regular Pilates practice will develop your self-awareness, helping you improve the way you go about your chores and reducing the strain they can put on your body. Try some of the exercises in this section the next time you feel manual tasks taking their toll on your body.

exercises for housework and DIY

- Pilates Squats
- Floating Arms
- Side Reach – Standing
- Waist Twist – Standing

Gardening

Gardening is a very popular pastime and, like any manual task, can put our bodies under pressure. The constant bending, stooping and kneeling involved affect the back, hips and knees, while the heavier tasks like digging and carrying can cause additional problems around the neck and shoulder region. A general Pilates session will offset any potential problems and the exercises in this section will help you release tension and keep you working from a strong centre when working in the garden.

Fishing

Although fishing often involves sitting for long periods of time, the actions of casting a line and reeling in a fish can be very physical. The area under most pressure is the back, due to the twisting and lifting motions, but when trying to land a fish, the forces on the arms and shoulders can also put these areas under strain. In between bites, try some of the exercises in the sedentary lifestyle section (page 262) to keep your body tension-free. Also practise the exercises in this section to help maintain strength and mobility in your spine, along with freedom of movement in the arms and shoulders.

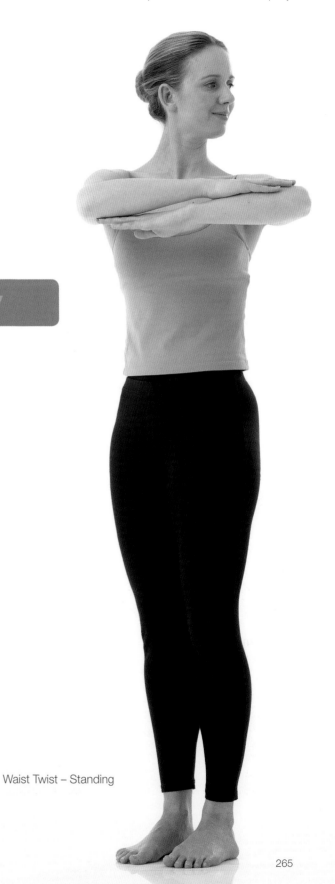

Waist Twist – Standing

Pilates at the gym

Most gym training is divided into two sections: cardiovascular training and resistance training. Generally, cardiovascular training is performed on fixed equipment like exercise bikes, treadmills, rowing machines and cross trainers. The main purpose of such activity is to exercise the heart and lungs, as well as build stamina in the muscles performing the exercise. Resistance training is usually performed on specialised machines, or with free weights such as barbells and dumbbells. The purpose of resistance training can vary from developing muscle strength to increasing muscular endurance; it can also give aesthetic benefits such as improved muscle tone or increased size and bulk.

We have included a selection of Pilates exercises that offer a great warm-up for any gym workout, but the real benefits lie in carrying the Pilates principles you have learnt into your regular gym exercises.

the pilates warm-up

exercises for pilates warm-up

- Knee Rolls
- Ribcage Closure
- Knee Folds
- Spine Curls
- Hip Rolls
- Curl Ups

- Single Leg Stretch – Preparation
- Dart
- The Cat
- Table Top
- Rest Position
- Zigzags – Sitting

- Roll Backs
- Side Reach – Standing
- Waist Twists – Standing
- Roll Downs

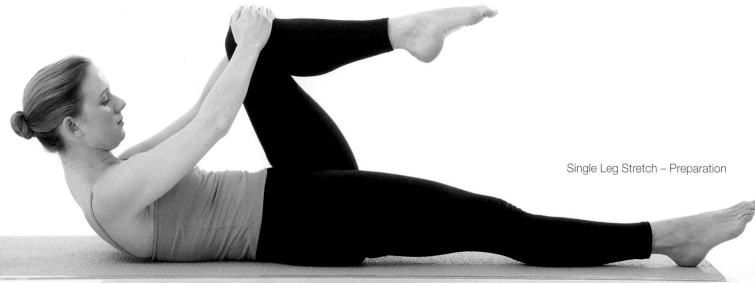

Single Leg Stretch – Preparation

a pilates focus for cardiovascular training

The Stationary Bike

Stationary bikes are very popular as they give the impression that you can sit down and still get fit! This is where the problems start. You will see people in gyms the world over, pedalling away while watching TV or chatting to friends, barely breaking a sweat and blissfully unaware of how poorly they are sitting, let alone how they are moving. Some gyms now offer bikes with workstations that allow you to surf the net and play games, which only add to the problem. Apart from the fact that the cardiovascular benefits are likely to be minimal, the other worrying thing is the potential damage that can be caused by exercising with poor movement quality. Just as in any Pilates session, you should engage the mind and the body to the same task; concentration and precision of movement are just as important here as they are performing the Single Leg Stretch! The challenge is to keep it up for 10–20 minutes.

POINTS TO FOCUS ON:

★ Set-up and sitting correctly

The height of the seat is the most important thing to consider when setting up the bike for you. When you are seated your heel should just reach the pedal, so when you bring the ball of your foot onto the pedal your knee is slightly bent. If you are too high, your pelvis will be forced to move from side to side and your knee will lock out. If you are too low, your knees will be bending too deeply, putting more strain on the front of the thighs and the knee joint, and your pelvis will tuck under on one side every time your knee comes up.

★ Upper body

Your shoulders should remain open and relaxed: avoid collapsing in between your shoulders or pressing too hard into the arms and rounding your shoulders as a result. Try to maintain length in your head and neck. Think of the open feeling in the front of the shoulders when doing the Dumb Waiter (page 82).

★ Leg alignment

The legs need to maintain good alignment throughout the pedalling action, your thigh bones, knees, shins, ankles and feet all working up and down in the same line from your hips. Think of Leg Slides.

★ Working both legs at the same time all the time

The most common mistake in the pedalling action is to push only down. Try to keep both legs working in opposing directions to one another at all times. Think of Single Leg Stretch (page 100).

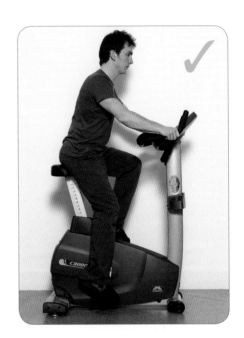

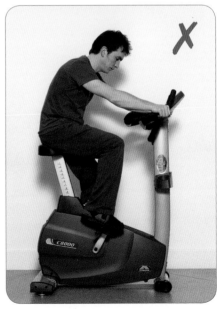

The Treadmill

The treadmill is another very popular piece of gym equipment as it offers flat, even running and walking in dry conditions 365 days a year. This said, many people are quite nervous using the treadmill at first as it is unlike most other bits of equipment in that it is actually moving you. For this very reason it provides quite a different experience from running or walking for real. Normally, if you were fatiguing while running or walking, you would reduce your speed automatically. However, on a treadmill you have consciously to tell the machine to slow down, which most people don't do when they need to. This leads to a compromised running or walking technique which often includes holding on with the arms. This is potentially quite damaging and serves no purpose; simply working at a manageable speed would give the same if not greater challenge to the cardiovascular system while maintaining good dynamic alignment and movement quality.

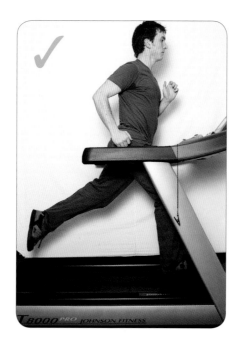

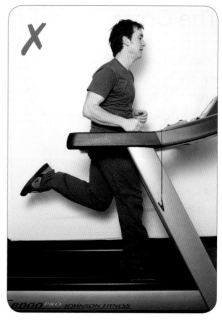

POINTS TO FOCUS ON:

★ **Speed**

Always run or walk at the right speed for you; it should feel that you are running the machine rather than the machine running you.

★ **Incline**

Avoid steep inclines, particularly when walking. These play havoc with good alignment and movement quality. Keep the incline under 5 per cent when walking and if you feel that you are unable to work hard enough, try running or maybe change to a cross trainer instead if you need to keep the activity low-impact.

★ **Alignment**

Stay tall and be as light-footed as you possibly can. Try thinking of any of your standing Pilates exercises: keep your neck lengthened and head balanced on top of your spine; your shoulders relaxed and your arms swinging freely with the walking and running action; your hips open and

released; and both halves of your body moving as symmetrically as possible.

★ **Breathing**

Your breath plays an important role in keeping your movement flowing and comfortable. If your breathing rhythm isn't attuned with your running or walking rhythm, you will become tense and restricted in your breathing or your technique – either way efficiency is compromised and tension-related discomfort will kick in. You will doubtless have suffered from a stitch in the past. Next time you do, try to notice which foot lands as you finish your out-breath, then try to change it to the other foot – it might help! Better still, try running or walking with an odd stride count so that the foot landing at the end of each out-breath is constantly alternating. Try also to adopt the controlled lateral breathing used in your Pilates exercises to regulate and pace your breathing volume and speed. You might just find you feel less fatigued.

The Cross Trainer

Cross trainers come in various shapes and sizes and are based on the mechanics of cross-country skiing. They provide a great cardiovascular exercise choice because, as when running you are weight-bearing through your legs and your arms are also actively employed with handles that move back and forth in time with the cyclical action of the legs. The added benefit for many over running is the low-impact nature of the movement which means that there are fewer issues arising from jarring forces. However, like many pieces of exercise equipment, cross trainers are often built around the average user's proportions with a limited amount of adjustability. Because these machines work through a set range of movement it is important that your body can follow this range without being pulled or pushed beyond its own range of movement. Try always to stand on and hold the handles in a way that allows your legs and arms to move freely with the minimum amount of disturbance to the lie of your body, neck and head.

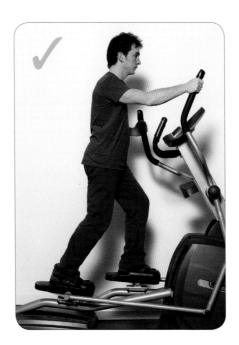

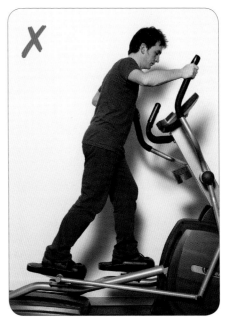

POINTS TO FOCUS ON:

★ **Speed**

Always work at manageable speeds. Although these machines are powered by you, they usually have heavy moving parts which, once in motion, get carried along by their own momentum, making sudden changes in speed difficult. Working from a strong centre will help you speed up and slow down with control and limit any jarring from the machine.

★ **Alignment**

Stay tall and try thinking of any of your standing Pilates exercises: keep your neck lengthened and head balanced on top of your spine; your shoulders relaxed and your arms moving freely with leg action; your hips open and released; and both halves of your body moving as symmetrically as possible.

★ **Breathing**

Your breath plays an important role in keeping your movement flowing and comfortable. If your breathing rhythm isn't attuned with the movement, you will become tense and restricted in your breathing or your technique and, either way, efficiency will be compromised. Try to use the controlled lateral breathing of your Pilates exercises to regulate and pace your breathing volume and speed. You might just find you feel less fatigued.

The Stepper or Climbing Machine

Similar to the treadmill and cross trainer, the stepper is a weight-bearing machine and requires good spinal alignment to be maintained while the legs (and arms on climbers) move up and down freely. Try to keep your head, back and pelvis balanced in the middle of the machine and work the legs from the hips, knees and ankles.

a pilates focus for resistance training machines

Resistance training with machines is a simple and effective way of training with resistance and works in much the same way as using Pilates studio equipment in that the closed chain nature of the exercises provides you with support and feedback throughout. Simply applying thoughtful techniques to many of these apparatus can make a huge difference to the effectiveness and safety of the exercises being performed.

One of the most limiting factors of resistance-training

machines is their fixed range of motion which doesn't allow the joint stability to be challenged appropriately during the movement. Apart from the fact that this enables you to 'cheat' the movement, it also gives you the potential to develop strength without the stability to control it. This is a recipe for disaster and increases the risk of injury over time. For this reason we highly recommend that, where available, you use equipment that uses cables and pulleys, thereby allowing multidirectional movement.

Leg Press

The Leg Press is essentially the same movement as the Footwork on the studio Reformer (page 170). The main differences are the amount of resistance being used and the full support of the feet on a foot plate rather than the partial support on a bar. Again, too much weight is the biggest cause of poor technique. As well as the direct comparison with the Footwork exercises on the Reformer, try to bear in mind what you have learnt from the following exercises:

- Pilates Squats (page 80)
- Leg Slides (page 31)
- Table Top (page 56)

.

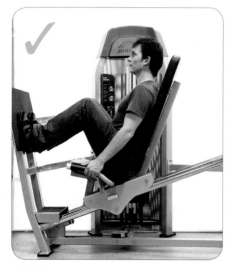 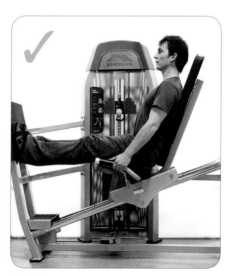 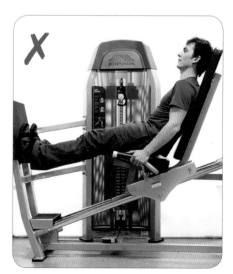

START   FINISH

Shoulder Press

The Shoulder Press movement is a challenging movement for the shoulder girdle to manage, especially when loaded with resistance. It also significantly challenges spinal alignment. If the exercise is performed with good-quality movements, you will not require too much resistance to get the training effect you are after. Try to think of what you have learnt from the following exercises:

- Ribcage Closure (page 37)
- Windows (page 51)
- Floating Arms (page 55)

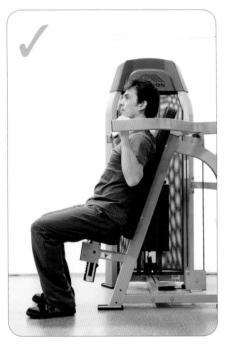

START

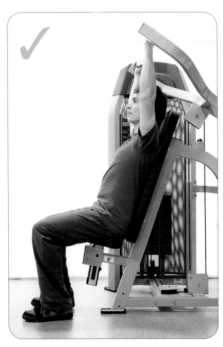

FINISH

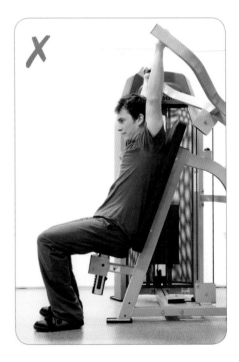

Lat Pulldown

The Lat Pulldown is effectively the same movement as the Shoulder Press but with the resistance being applied on the way down rather than on the way up. It is less stressful for the shoulder girdle with the load of resistance but still presents a significant challenge to your spinal alignment. Many exercises try to pass the bar behind the head which will almost always cause alignment issues. For this reason we recommend sitting back slightly and pulling the bar in front of the head. Again, movement quality should always be prioritised over resistance. Try to think of what you have learnt from the following exercises:

- Ribcage Closure (page 37)
- Windows (page 51)
- Floating Arms (page 55)

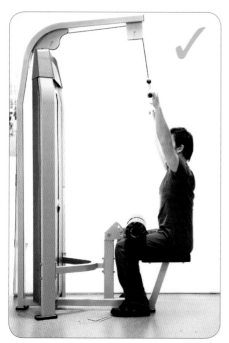

START

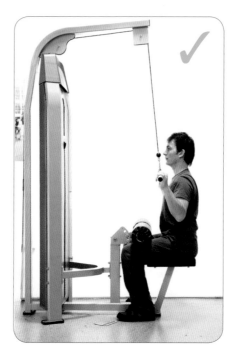

FINISH

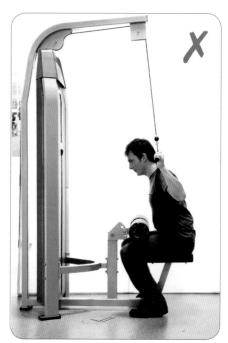

Chest Press

The Chest Press movement is a challenging one for the shoulder girdle to manage, especially when loaded with resistance. The challenge for spinal alignment comes entirely from bad technique, with people often arching their lower backs to cope with a resistance that is too heavy. If the exercise is performed with good-quality movements, you will not require as much resistance as you might think to get the training effect you are after. Try to think of what you have learnt from the following exercises:

- Windows (page 51)
- Flys (page 229)
- Bow and Arrow – Sitting (page 60)

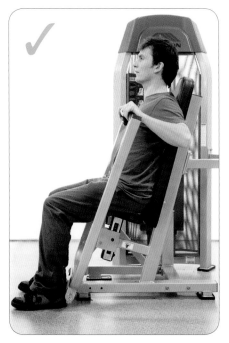

START

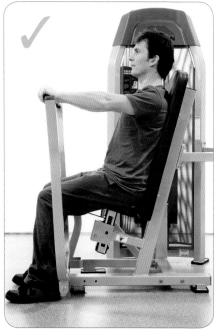

FINISH

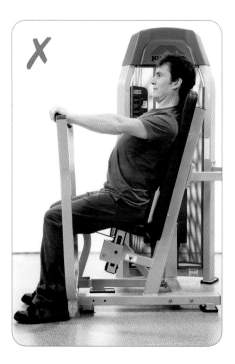

Seated Row

The Seated Row exercise is a similar movement to the Chest Press except that the resistance is pulled in towards the body rather than being pressed away. It is not over-stressful for the shoulder girdle and the challenge to your spinal alignment is usually fairly manageable if there is a chest pad to support the body's position. If there isn't, the role of supporting the seated position is passed to the back muscles and legs. However, swinging into an arched back position is likely if it is too heavy.

Again, movement quality should always be prioritised over resistance. Try to think of what you have learnt from the following exercises:

- Windows (page 51)
- Flys (page 229)
- Bow and Arrow – Sitting (page 60)

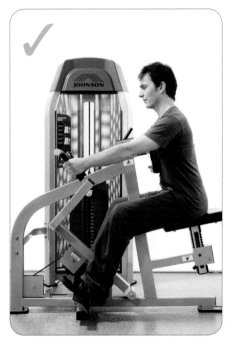

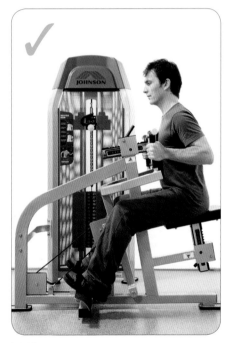

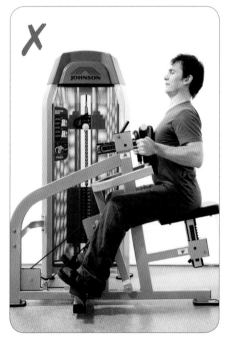

START

FINISH

a pilates focus for free-weight resistance training

Resistance training with free weights is a more challenging way of training with resistance and works in a similar way to Pilates matwork in that the exercises challenge the body with gravity and offer much less support and feedback throughout. The fact that there is resistance involved means poor technique can be extremely damaging to the joints and soft tissue surrounding them. Applying the same thoughtful approach to alignment and technique as you do in a Pilates session is fundamental to safe effective use of free weights. We have selected five commonly used free-weight exercises to give you an idea of how to apply what you have learnt in your Pilates sessions to your free-weight resistance training.

Bench/Chest Press

The Bench Press movement is traditionally performed with a barbell, although dumbbells can also be used (hence the exercise is sometimes known as Dumbbell Chest Press) are actually more effective as they offer a greater challenge to the stability of the shoulder while strengthening the chest and shoulder area. The stability of the shoulders is the key thing to focus on here – working with too much resistance will result in this being compromised. The challenge for spinal alignment is a result of bad technique, people often arching their lower backs to cope with a resistance that is too heavy. Try to think of what you have learnt from the following exercises:

- Windows (page 51)
- Flys (page 229)
- Bow and arrow – Sitting (page 60)

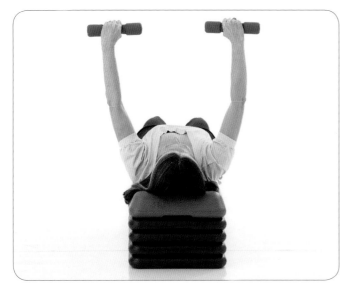

START

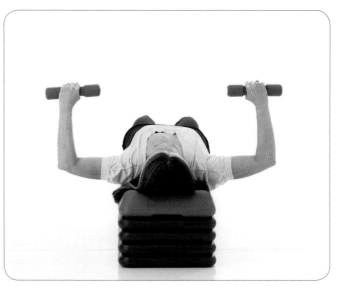

FINISH

Flys

The Fly is a favourite for developing strength and tone across the chest. It is important to keep open across the chest during the exercise and again not to work with too much resistance. Stability of the shoulder girdle should not be compromised as the leverage on the joint is high and therefore increases the risk of injury. Spinal stability also needs to be maintained throughout. If the exercise is performed with good-quality movements, you will not require as much resistance as you might think to get the training effect you are after. Try to think of what you have learnt from the following exercises:

- Flys (page 229)
- Windows (page 51)
- Arm Openings (page 64)

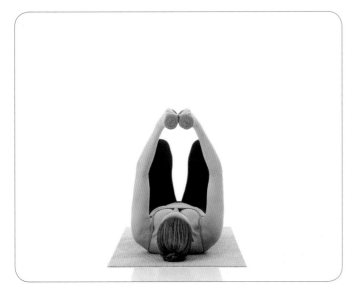

START

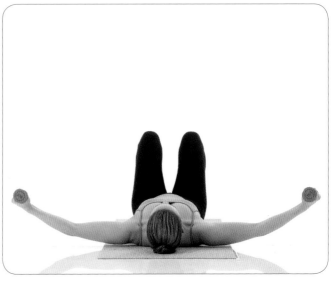

FINISH

Lateral Raises

This is a great exercise for developing the muscles around the shoulder girdle and is a very popular choice for gym users. However, techniques can vary dramatically – many of them are potentially harmful to the neck and shoulder area. As always, quality of movement is the most important factor to consider when performing the exercise. You will definitely not require as much resistance to get the training effect you are after if you maintain a well-balanced technique. Try to think of what you have learnt from the following exercises:

- Floating Arms (page 55)
- Ribcage Closure (page 37)
- Windows (page 51)

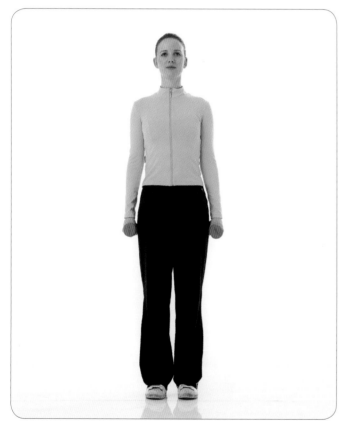

START

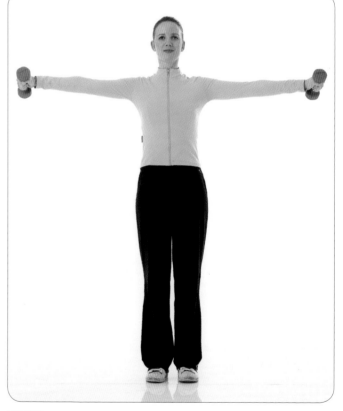

FINISH

Squats

There are various types of Squat exercise requiring different bar positions and ranges of movement. Wherever the bar is placed, it often proves very difficult to organise good spinal alignment, particularly if the range of movement at the shoulders is restricted. Although the spine's alignment will compensate to a degree, it is important not to allow it to move too far from neutral alignment during the movement, or use the dumbbell version as shown here. Try to think of what you have learnt from the following exercises:

- Sliding Down the Wall with the Big Ball (page 218)
- Pilates Squats (page 80)
- Arm Openings (page 64)

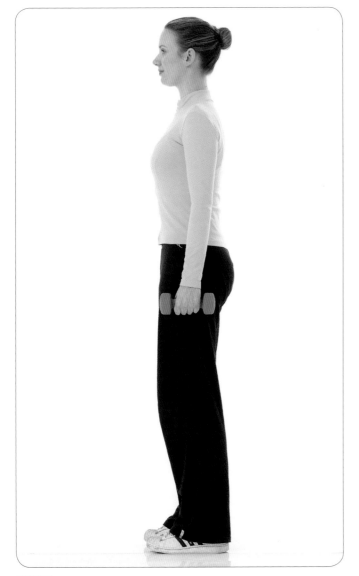

START

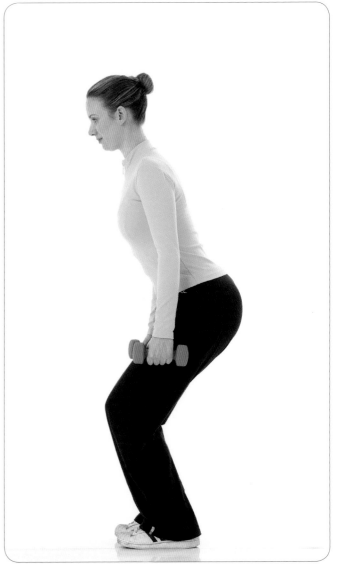

FINISH

Lunges

There are various types of lunging exercises working through various ranges of movement and directions. With the bar behind the head it is difficult to organise good spinal alignment, particularly if your shoulders are tight. The version we have shown here is the backwards lunge as this makes it easier to maintain good alignment and control. Try to maintain neutral alignment during the movement and think of what you have learnt from the following exercises:

- Standing Leg Press with the Band (page 195)
- Pilates Squats (page 80)
- Table Top (page 56)

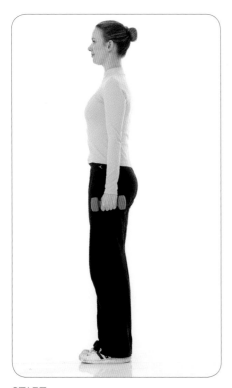

START

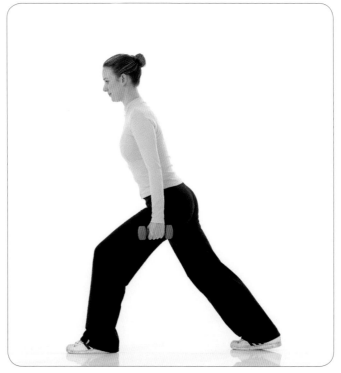

FINISH

Pilates for sports

Pilates for Running

Running is the most natural of all physical activities as our bodies are designed for it. All that is required is suitable footwear and the great outdoors and away you go. It is an excellent way to keep in shape, exercising your heart and lungs and toning the whole body. The main issues usually arise from poor technique, which Pilates can certainly help improve. The following exercises are recommended:

- Spine Curls
- Hip Rolls
- Curl Ups
- Single Leg Stretch – Preparation
- Cobra Prep
- Single Leg Kicks
- Roll Downs
- Pilates Squats

Pilates for Cycling

Cycling is growing increasingly popular as more and more people chose the bike over the car to get to and from work or for outings at the weekend. Technique and bike set-up are extremely important. We would always recommend you to consult your local bike shop for advice on what sort of bike is appropriate for you and to ask them to set it up specifically for you. The seated position adopted when riding does compromise your spinal alignment quite significantly. This is particularly the case when riding performance road and mountain bikes. Regular Pilates sessions will help offset time spent in the saddle and help improve the efficiency of your riding technique. Try:

- Knee Rolls
- Spine Curls
- Single Leg Stretch
- Diamond Press
- Star
- Single Leg Kick
- Table Top
- The Cat

Pilates for Swimming

Swimming is a great full-body activity, exercising your heart and lungs and helping improve muscle tone throughout the whole body. Recreationally, there is a very low incidence of problems, thanks to the support and feedback provided by the surrounding water. The problems that do arise usually result from poor technique and overuse. Pilates can help keep your body's movements balanced which helps you refine your swimming technique. The following exercises should prove helpful:

- Shoulder Drops
- Arm Circles
- Oblique Curl Ups
- The Cat
- Table Top
- Double Leg Kick
- Swimming
- Roll Downs

Pilates for Rowing

Rowing is physically demanding whatever your level. It really is a full-body movement, requiring a good range of movement in all of your joints. As with so many activities the importance of technique is paramount to staying injury-free. That said, the mechanical movements performed in the rowing action are particularly challenging for the body's natural biomechanics to cope with. Given that this action is performed hundreds of times in a session, it is particularly important to counter all this work with movements in other directions. Pilates provides an excellent supplement to your rowing training, giving your body a chance to rebalance and maintain its ability to keep performing time and time again. Try the following exercises:

- Roll Downs
- Pilates Squats
- Zigzags – Sitting
- Spine Stretch Forward
- Side Reach – Sitting
- Waist Twist – Sitting
- Cobra
- The Cat

Pilates for Sailing and Windsurfing

Both sailing and windsurfing test the whole body, often in extremely challenging conditions. There is a lot of upper body work required in both disciplines, much of it with the arms overhead. This challenges not only the arms and shoulders, but also the stability of the back. This coupled with the fact that movements have to be performed reactively to the situation and are multidirectional, means the demands on the body can be quite intense. All Pilates exercises will therefore have a positive effect on your performance and help keep you injury-free, including the following:

- Windows
- Spine Curls
- Oblique Curl Ups
- The Cat
- Table Top
- Bow and Arrow – Sitting
- Spine Stretch Forward
- Roll Downs

Pilates for Skiing and Snowboarding

By far the most popular activity-holiday choices, skiing and snowboarding can be quite physically demanding. Not least because most people do it for only one or two weeks of the year, so the body is often ill-prepared for the sudden change of use. Even if you ski or board all season, your body still needs adequate time to prepare for the demands it faces on the slopes. The biggest physical challenge is to the legs and lower back. However, if you are a beginner, you will often spend a lot of your time picking yourself up from the ground. This will also require a lot of work in those arms and upper back, so a well-balanced Pilates routine is an ideal solution in the weeks leading up to a trip. These exercises should help:

- The Cat
- Table Top
- Zigzags – Sitting
- Knee Rolls
- Spine Curls
- Single Leg Stretch
- Double Leg Stretch
- Pilates Squats

Pilates for Team Sports

Whether you play at professional or amateur level, team sports like football, rugby, cricket and hockey place enormous demands on the body. They are fast-paced and require sudden changes of direction and pace along with kicking, throwing and jumping actions. This means that players are at risk of strain-related injuries to their muscles, tendons and joints. Players therefore need to stay mobile and agile as well as strong and powerful. Developing the dynamic stability needed to control all that power at speed is something Pilates exercises can really help with. Try the following:

- Spine Curls
- Knee Rolls
- Oblique Curl Ups
- Single Leg Stretch – Preparation
- Cobra Prep
- Single Leg Kicks
- The Cat
- Roll Downs

Pilates for Tennis and other Racquet Sports

Tennis requires agility and mobility coupled with precision and focus. The quality and control of spinal and upper-limb movement are fundamental to good technique. Pilates exercises will really help improve this, through the awareness and self-control it develops. The repetitive and forceful nature of the movements involved in the game also brings risk of strain in and around the joints of the arm. Pilates exercises will also help to keep the balance between stability and mobility at an optimal level around these joints. Practising regular Pilates sessions in between matches as part of your regular training will really help you stay on top of your game; incorporate the following exercises:

- Waist Twist – Standing
- Side Reach – Standing
- Oblique Curl Ups
- Single Leg Stretch – Preparation
- Cobra Prep
- Single Leg Kicks
- Roll Downs
- Pilates Squats

Pilates for Golf

Golf is a relatively slow-paced sport. However, the powerful and repetitive swing action required puts quite a strain on the back, arms and shoulders. Poor technique can contribute too many of the aches and pains that often arise from playing regularly. The perfect swing requires a high degree of mobility as well as precision and power. This is often overlooked by many golfers who continue to try to build their technique on the shaky foundations of poor body mechanics. Taking time out from the driving range to practise Pilates, even once a week, could dramatically improve your game by developing your movement potential. It will also help you stave off strain-related injuries. The following exercises are recommended:

- Hip Rolls
- Oblique Curl Ups
- Arm Openings
- Single Leg Kicks
- Roll Downs
- Waist Twist – Standing
- Side Reach – Standing
- Pilates Squats

Pilates for Horse Riding

Horse riding of any kind and at any level demands a high degree of balance and control. Many riding injuries are the result of falls. Regular Pilates will help your riding on many levels; principally the improvements it will make to your core strength will help your riding technique and increase your endurance in the saddle. It will also help increase the mobility in your hips, keep your shoulders released and improve your spinal alignment and posture, all important qualities of good riding technique. Try the following exercises:

- Double Knee Folds
- Spine Curls
- Hip Rolls
- Seated C-Curve
- Zigzags – Sitting
- Waist Twist – Sitting
- Dart
- The Cat

Pilates for Dance and Gymnastics

Dance and gymnastics both demand high levels of physical development, agility, control and precision of movement. Pilates is an ideal accompaniment to the training sessions for either discipline. Indeed, many dance schools include Pilates in the curriculum for this very reason. The biggest problem faced by dancers and gymnasts when doing Pilates exercises is that their bodies are usually well suited to doing these sorts of movements already, making even the hardest Pilates exercises look and feel easy. However, this is exactly why Pilates is so useful, as what is essential is the way the exercises are performed. While dancers and gymnasts may look as though they are doing an exercise well, they often end up working from the wrong muscles and 'cheating' the movements. Therefore it is important to spend time on the lower-level exercises in order to feel how the movement comes from somewhere deeper. All the exercises in this book have relevance to either activity, helping you gain more core control and fine tuning the way that you move, but here is a selection to work on:

- Spine Curls
- Double Leg Stretch – Preparation
- Roll Ups
- Zigzags – Sitting
- Spine Twist
- Mermaid
- Cobra
- Roll Downs

Further Information

Body Control Pilates is headquartered in Bloomsbury in the heart of London, where we operate studios and public classes as well as running our teacher-training and development courses. We also have training partners in countries as diverse as Canada, Denmark, Norway, Portugal and South Africa. Our membership body has become Europe's largest professional Pilates organisation, with all certified Body Control Pilates teachers having, at a minimum, completed a comprehensive training course in Body Control Pilates matwork and thereafter working to a laid-down Code of Practice governing teaching standards, professional ethics and continuing education. This ensures that our teachers continue to build their own skills and knowledge on a regular basis.

PILATES INFORMATION AND TEACHERS
Body Control Pilates Association
www.bodycontrol.co.uk
www.bodycontrolpilates.com
Pilates World University
www.pilatesworlduniversity.com

UK REGISTER OF EXERCISE PROFESSIONALS
www.exerciseregister.org

PILATES HOME ACCESSORIES
Body Control Pilates website
www.bodycontrol.co.uk
Foam Rollers (Fit Roll)
www.sisseluk.com

PHYSIOTHERAPY
Charted Society of Physiotherapists
www.csp.org.uk
Chartered Physiotherapists in Women's Health
www.acpwh.org.uk

CHIROPRACTIC
General Chiropractic Council
www.gcc-uk.org

OSTEOPATHY
General Osteopathic Council
www.osteopathy.org.uk

National Back Pain Association UK
Back Care
www.backcare.org.uk

PILATES FOR GOLF
Courses for golfers at all levels
www.bodycontrolpilatesgolf.com

BOOKS
Pilates for Weight Loss
Lynne Robinson
(Kyle Cathie)

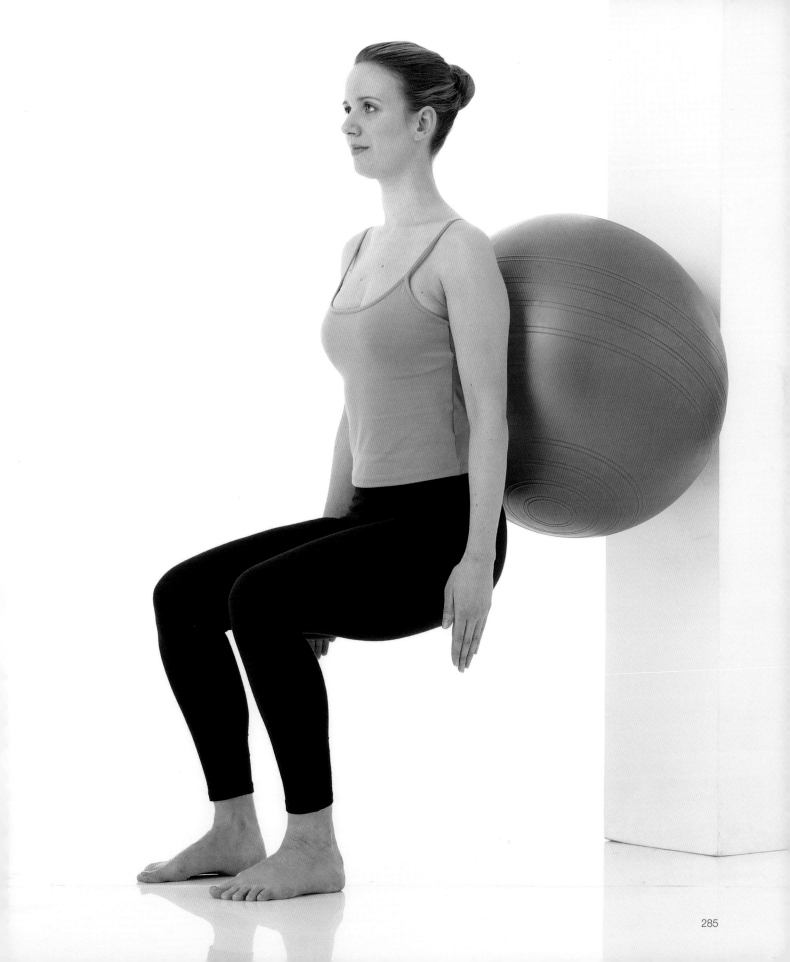

index

acknowledgements

Lynne Robinson

When we founded Body Control Pilates back in 1995, we knew we had created an approach to teaching Pilates that was new and exciting, we knew it had potential, but we could not possibly have known that it would grow to become such a huge international success.

Looking back over that time, I have watched our method evolve and our Body Control Pilates community develop into something unique. This growth has been due to the skills and dedication of our teachers; to the hard work and commitment of the staff at our London Centre (my thanks especially to Tim), and last, but by no means least, to the inspiration we draw from the many thousands of clients who believe in the Body Control Pilates approach. I cannot name you all, but I can thank you all.

A special thanks to our fabulous medical consultant Kate Fernyhough, Chartered Physiotherapist and Body Control Pilates teacher, who, once again, kindly read through our manuscript and offered her invaluable advice.

Rarely for me, I'm struggling now to find the right words to express the depth of my gratitude to my co-authors Lisa and Nathan. Writing a book of this magnitude is no easy task. It requires not just exceptional talent as Pilates teachers, but also a vision for the future. Lisa and Nathan, thanks to you, I believe that the best is still to come…

Lisa Bradshaw

This book is a collaboration of many people's work and I certainly could not have contributed if it were not for the support of my colleagues and friends. First I must thank the Robinsons, Leigh and Lynne, for always having faith in me and for giving me a platform to do the work that I love. They have been supportive and steadfast throughout and for that I am very grateful.

My thanks go also to Nathan Gardner and Sarah Marks who have consistently been my allies for the past few years; it is not only their expertise but also their determination, focus and good humour that have allowed our work to develop. I hope that this can continue for many years to come.

I have had many teachers in the past to whom I am eternally grateful; in particular Heather and Martin Samson, who opened up the world of Pilates to me and set me graciously on my initial journey. It is, however, the clients and students that I have worked with over the years who have taught, inspired and encouraged me to continue exploring; in particular I would like to thank Sarah for giving me the confidence to be the teacher that I am; Jill for showing me on a daily basis that the body is such a fascinating and miraculous tool that just keeps on improving; and Prue, who taught me with a little bit of Pilates and a lot of tenacity we can surely overcome many of the obstacles in our lives.

On a personal note a huge thank you must go to my family who have simply always been there, smiling and supporting my every decision. Finally the biggest thanks of all must go to Lee, my greatest cheerleader and most respected critic. With your patience and strength, how could I fail? Thank you always.

Nathan Gardner

My primary thanks must of course go to my fellow authors, Lynne and Lisa, who have been incredibly upbeat and focused throughout this entire project. As work colleagues we have worked closely together for a number of years now and this project has just reinforced what can be achieved with open-mindedness and mutual respect. I must also extend this thank you to Sarah Marks who has worked consistently alongside us over the years as part of our team, helping build and develop the educational programme here at Body Control Pilates.

I would like to say thank you to our photographer Eddie who worked tirelessly behind the camera and whose expertise and professionalism have ensured that the images in this book look fantastic. Equally a big thank you must go to his subjects, our additional Pilates models, Marie, Bridget and Samir, all of whom are fantastic teachers in their own right. There are many other people who have helped make this book a reality: thanks to you all.

Finally, to the colleagues, clients and friends and in particular my loved ones, present and departed, who have inspired and supported me over the years, I would like to say a very special thank you.